# DOWN SYNDROME AND VITAMIN THERAPY

## UNLOCKING THE SECRETS OF IMPROVED HEALTH, BEHAVIOUR AND INTELLIGENCE

by **Kent MacLeod**

FOREWORD BY
DR. ABRAM HOFFER M.D. PH.D.

WITHDRAWN FROM LIBRARY
BRITISH MEDICAL ASSOCIATION

D1427701

1004714

# ACKNOWLEDGEMENTS

To my wife, Linda Pollon. Without her ongoing work, support, love and leadership I could never have completed this project. I humbly offer my love as poor compensation for her efforts and patience.

To Kim Pittaway my wonderful editor. Thank you for editing and applying your amazing writing and organizing skills to this book.

To Dr. Abe Hoffer, and Dr. Bernie Rimland. For years they have been dedicated to a healthier approach to mental issues in spite of the obstacles. My struggles pale in comparison to their years of dedication.

To Roger Biddle, thank you for your advice and encouragement.

To all my incredible staff who have been so dedicated and hard working... thank you.

Most importantly a heartfelt thanks to all the parents. Each day I am simply in awe of the tremendous courage and love they bring to their children. I am pulled and pushed by these incredible parents with every meeting and every phone call. If I can make their lives and the lives of their children better by any measure with this book then I will have succeeded.

ACQUISITION

# TABLE OF CONTENTS

# TABLE OF CONTENTS

# TABLE OF CONTENTS

# TABLE OF CONTENTS

# FOREWORD

## BY DR. ABRAM HOFFER, M.D., PH.D.

---

**INTRODUCTION TO DR. HOFFER**

*by Kent MacLeod*

*There are very few physicians in the world today who deserve more credit for establishing the value of vitamins, minerals and other nutrients than Dr. Abram Hoffer. His pioneering contribution to the rapidly expanding field of nutritional medicine over the past 50 years is known internationally through his more than 500 publications and extensive lecturing.*

*At age 85, Dr. Hoffer is as sharp as most of his colleagues half his age. He still works four days per week at his clinic in Victoria, British Columbia, and is always preparing new publications and lectures. His practice, which began primarily as psychiatric, has evolved to include hundreds of cancer patients referred to him by their oncologists. Says Hoffer, "They usually come to me when their doctors have exhausted the possibilities of standard treatment. Just imagine how well they'd be if they sought orthomolecular treatment first!"*

*Dr. Hoffer founded the American Schizophrenia Association (later known as the Huxly Institute for Biosocial Research) in 1964, and the Canadian Schizophrenia Foundation in 1968. One of Dr. Hoffer's many books,* How to Live with Schizophrenia, *attracted the attention of two-time Nobel Laureate Linus Pauling who coined the word orthomolecular in his seminal paper published in* Science *in 1968. Hoffer's work had a significant* influence on Pauling who joined the editorial board of the Journal of Orthomolecular Psychiatry. *This respected publication, which Hoffer founded in 1972, was renamed the* Journal of Orthomolecular Medicine *in 1986. Together, Hoffer and Pauling published important studies showing the positive effects of orthomolecular treatment for cancer.*

*Through five decades as a practising physician and researcher, Abram Hoffer has experienced the slow shifting of attitudes regarding nutritional medicine. He has never lost his courageous vision or his remarkable receptivity to new ideas.*

I first became interested in Down Syndrome when I heard about the work being done by Dr. Henry Turkel in Detroit many years ago. He developed a multivitamin, multimineral preparation with thyroid which he gave to a large number of children with Down Syndrome and he consistently reported good to excellent results. I published many of his papers in the *Journal of Orthomolecular Psychiatry* and its earlier versions. Dr. Turkel suffered the fate of almost all early pioneers. He had the nerve to make his claims when everyone "knew" that children with genetic defects could not possibly be treated successfully. He fought back with great ferocity but at last was restricted to shipping his product only in Michigan with major penalties if he were to send it across the Michigan border to any other place. Eventually he retired to Israel. He bequeathed his books to Dr. Bernard Rimland who has been distributing them. I have a couple of copies. Apparently the treatment is much more popular in Japan.

> The best way to have a good idea is to have lots of ideas.
> – Linus Pauling

Over the ensuing years, there appeared to be little progress in the area of nutritional treatments for children with Down Syndrome, probably because American physicians were too fearful of the FDA and their own parent organizations to try it. Then Kent MacLeod started his clinical studies and his laboratory.

This book is the outcome of his work over the past 20 years. Using the most modern laboratory tests, MacLeod and his group analyze the abnormal biochemistry of children with Down Syndrome, as well as other children who might have Autism or one of the attention deficit syndromes. When the abnormal pathology is detected and corrected with the correct use of the nutrients these children improve. They are not cured in the same way that diabetes is never cured. With diabetes the patients must take insulin and watch their food forever. The same holds true for Down Syndrome: they must take their special nutrient formula and watch their diet forever. This is a small price to pay for the health improvements that come from this program.

MacLeod provides many case histories of children and their families on the pages that follow.

One must give credit to the parents, especially the mothers, who fight so hard and search so diligently for information which will help their children recover. They had to face the usual opposition from a profession which still believes that nutrients are of little value and that nothing can be done. These cases are very convincing. If I had a Down Syndrome child I would immediately consult Kent MacLeod. I wish he lived in Victoria B.C. rather than in Ottawa.

MacLeod uses orthomolecular treatment. This word, coined by Linus Pauling in 1968, has become increasingly popular as physicians realize what it means for their patients. It emphasizes the use of organic molecules that are normally present in the body. It does not include the use of herbs or drugs but these are useful in some cases as adjuncts to the main therapy. When the biochemical abnormalities are corrected with the right nutrients in optimum doses the disease comes under control. In the case of children with Down Syndrome, the children gain the intelligence their genes have organized for them, their behaviour becomes normal, they become productive and they do not suffer the stigma of chronic disease. The improved health and productivity that results for each child probably saves the country in which they live and their parents $2 million over their natural life span of between 45 and 50 years.

This book provides useful descriptions of the many nutrients which may be involved and how they are used. In my opinion this treatment approach must be used for all of these children. One day it will be, when medical schools in Canada wake up and start teaching its method. I suppose they are still waiting for double blind randomized therapeutic trials that no drug company will fund because the treatment can not be patented.

A. HOFFER M.D., PH.D. FRCP(C)

# NUTRI-CHEM'S BEGINNINGS

As a scientist you don't just wake up one morning and decide to follow a particular path of research and study. The starting point for my work with families of children with Down Syndrome began with a family crisis of my own. I was a third-year pharmacy student at the University of Toronto in Canada. My grandmother was dying of pancreatic cancer, cared for at home by family in Timmins, my hometown in northern Ontario.

As her cancer progressed, my grandmother became unable to swallow oral medications and relied on visits from her physician for morphine injections to relieve her pain. These weren't working, though, and my family turned to me – a pharmacy student and the first in my family to attend university – for help.

## WHAT WILL I LEARN?
Nutritional therapy can help your child

- have fewer infections
- have more vitality both physically and mentally
- and avoid debilitating diseases.

I'll never forget the call from my mother pleading for something to ease my grandmother's pain. Morphine suppositories would have been the answer, but at that time no drug company made them since the market wasn't profitable enough. I remember the feeling of impotence I had as I told my mother that nothing could be done.

After I graduated two years later and set up my pharmaceutical practice in Ottawa, I made morphine suppositories available in Canada. This was the start of my journey and my commitment to serving the needs of people who had been abandoned or ignored by conventional medicine or drug corporations. My approach was a simple one: "Solve the Problem."

My Ottawa pharmacy was non-traditional from the start. It quickly became a place people came to for solutions. I found that once I left the fold of the drug industry and focused on meeting people's needs, all kinds of doors opened, revealing new approaches that traditional physicians had either ignored or dismissed.

I had an extensive background in biochemistry and specialized in nutritional interventions for a variety of disorders. One of the doctors I worked with was interested in a nutritional approach to solving some of the problems her young patients were having that conventional drug therapies didn't help, such as antibiotics for recurring bronchitis. Some of these patients were children with Down Syndrome.

## One mother's question

In 1982, I met a mother who helped shape the direction of my work. This woman's young son was severely brain injured with seizures occurring several times each hour around the clock. Often these seizures were triggered by chemicals and dyes in foods and the very drugs that were supposed to be helping the boy. I customized his medication, tailoring it to his specific requirements but removing the dyes and additives.

At the same time, while researching this boy's condition and medication, I realized that vitamin B6 had a dramatic effect in stopping his seizures. The additive-free drugs, together with the B6, worked. His seizures stopped. Yet his mother had to battle an arrogant medical staff to administer vitamin B6 to her son. The medical staff refused to administer intravenous vitamin B6 to him even though it was safe and would stop his seizures. Instead they favoured more invasive and dangerous drug therapies.

From this experience, I became convinced of three things:

- nutrition can make a dramatic difference;
- we need to individualize compounds;
- the medical profession is reluctant to use vitamins even where there is a demonstrated benefit and no demonstrable harm.

This mother was excited about the beneficial results of the nutritional therapy on her son's development. Told by the medical profession that he would not live beyond the age of three or four, she was determined to prove them wrong. She began exploring how nutritional changes might benefit him and discovered the work on nutrients done by Dr. Henry Turkel of Michigan and Dr. Franz Schmid of Germany.

Dr. Turkel's formulation for children with Down Syndrome combined vitamins and minerals along with drugs such as nasal decongestants, diuretics and thyroid hormones. He made claims that his compound would improve intelligence and alter physical characteristics associated with Down Syndrome.

She asked me to take at look at the findings of Drs. Turkel and Schmid and comment on them. She set up a meeting with a small group of parents (one of whom was Eleanor Pinsonneault whose son Daniel is profiled in *Chapter One* in this book) who had children with Down Syndrome, and I shared my thoughts on Turkel's approach with them. Faced with the extravagant claims by Dr. Turkel as well as a desire to help their children, the parents in that original meeting asked two important questions:

- Will this cure my child? Will it do everything?
- Is this useless for my child? Will it do nothing?

# Nutrition supports health

The answer to both questions was no. Nutritional therapy adds a third dimension – called biological complementariness – to the traditional two-dimensional medical approach of risk versus benefit. With no risk involved, nutritional therapy looks at how to be supportive or essential to health. We're not talking about "curing" a disorder with genetic origins. Instead, we're looking at how children can have fewer infections, more vitality both physically and mentally, and avoid debilitating future diseases.

Nutrition is not an all-or-nothing phenomenon, and parents need to understand its limitations and its potential. Two nutritional laws are basic to this understanding:

- Synergy – all nutrients help each other and function interdependently;
- Completeness – if even one essential nutrient is deficient, there will be adverse health consequences.

At the meeting with the parents, I said that if I were considering this treatment for my child, I would change Turkel's formula. First, I would remove the drug components to make it safer. Then, I would improve the nutritional ingredients to make it safe and more effective.

"Then why don't you do it?" one woman quickly asked. I proceeded to develop the first MSB formula.

# Solutions for everyday problems and prevention for the future

The experience with these parents illustrates an important lesson: there are plenty of extravagant claims about the benefits of nutritional therapies, and unfortunately, those claims can do more harm than good. First, such claims obscure the more subtle but still real benefits of nutritional therapies. Second, they make all of us who believe in the benefits of nutritional therapies targets for those who are justifiably skeptical about over-the-top claims. And they make it easy for the skeptics to ignore the real benefits as they focus instead on the hype.

In my experience, parents are much smarter and more realistic than both those making over-the-top claims and the skeptics on the other side give them credit for. Parents of children with Down Syndrome know that, at this stage in our scientific development, a cure for those already born with Down Syndrome is nothing short of science fiction. But we can make a difference in the quality of life for those with Down Syndrome by addressing some of the symptoms associated with the disorder.

And that's what most parents are after: solutions for everyday problems today and prevention for the future. Nutritional therapy can make that difference.

## Extravagant claims

Our work with families of children with Down Syndrome continued to grow slowly with no attempt on our part to promote the use of vitamin supplements. Word spread, however, as parents told one another of the health benefits to their children. All this changed in 1995 when a Louisiana parent, Dixie Lawrence, appeared on national television in the U.S. claiming that nutritional therapy could raise I.Q. and alter physical attributes associated with Down Syndrome.

Dixie, whose adopted daughter, Madison, had Down Syndrome, had tracked down Dr. Henry Turkel in Israel after reading about his vitamin therapies. Dr. Turkel was retired and no longer practicing medicine, and told Dixie about our work at Nutri-Chem. She contacted me and asked if I would look at customizing our nutritional supplement based on her daughter's lab test results.

At this time, I became aware of work being done in France by Dr. Marie Peeters-Ney, a pediatric hemotologist, and Dr. Jerome Lejeune (discoverer of the cause of Down Syndrome). Their research on amino acid deficiencies in the genetic disorder linked to certain genes on the 21st chromosome, combined with the positive benefits reported by parents whose children had been taking our MSB supplement for 10 years, convinced me to work with Dixie on a customized formula for her daughter that incorporated Lejeune's and Peeters-Ney' research.

Excited about the beneficial results on her daughter Madison, Dixie began to talk about Nutri-Chem's MSB formula. She appeared on the U.S. network television program *Day One*, talking about the nutritional "therapy" that she said had raised Madison's I.Q. and changed some of her physical characteristics. Pitted against Dixie's claims were established medical researchers who disputed the benefits of nutritional therapy and warned against the "alternative charlatans" who were taking advantage of vulnerable parents, making money off their desire to improve their children's health. It made for good T.V. – concerned mother versus the medical establishment – and evoked a good deal of emotion. It also catapulted the issue of nutritional therapy for children with Down Syndrome onto the national scene.

Following the *Day One* program, Dixie gave our address to parents who contacted her after seeing the television program. Interest in Nutri-Chem's MSB formula exploded. Excited about the increased awareness and interest in nutritional therapy in Down syndrome, I felt, along with our researchers, that this was not an endpoint in our work, and that we should continue our understanding of the efficacy of nutritional therapies and focus on research and development to further improve the formula. You will note throughout this book references to our study and research projects.

## A consistent approach: solve the problem without harming the body

At Nutri-Chem, our approach and philosophy about nutritional therapies have remained consistent: treat the body's system as an integrated whole, separate fact from fantasy, and above all "solve the problem" without harming the body.

Like most parents, we view quality of life in all its facets as a measure of health. When a child has fewer upper respiratory infections, they lose less time to illness. Hearing, a crucial factor in language development, improves. Along with this we see better communication skills, a key indicator of intelligence. With increased nutrient absorption, growth and energy are enhanced resulting in more mental alertness and a greater ability to learn. Nutritional supplements improve immune system function, benefitting brain development and preventing premature aging and death of brain cells (the medical term for this is apoptosis). All of these things can contribute to enabling a child to function more fully to their potential.

Vitamin supplements improve immune function and reduce respiratory infections and ear infections. They increase energy and improve quality of life. But do they improve I.Q.?

The unequivocal answer is yes. While there is still research to be done in this area, new studies show that vitamin supplements have a positive effect on I.Q. The results are impressive enough to have become the cornerstone of a national program funded by the U.S. Congress and operated by the Healthy Foundation (www.healthfound.org), designed to provide free supplements to low-income children. While the studies have not been conducted on children with Down Syndrome, there's no reason to believe the results would not be true for children who are even more genetically vulnerable to vitamin and mineral deficiencies than the general public. (See *Chapter 3: Vitamins and Your Child's Intelligence* for more on this important topic.)

But even if I.Q. were not affected by vitamins, the simple fact is that better health will allow children with Down Syndrome to laugh, play, learn and interact more completely with the world around them. Add the benefits to I.Q., and the case for supplementation becomes even more persuasive.

## Treat the problem, not the Down Syndrome

Today, nutritional supplements are gaining wider acceptance for their ability to improve health, enhance quality of life, and prevent disease. There is growing awareness that many costly drug therapies often only mask the symptoms of disease or, as in the case of most prescribed antibiotics, they actually make people sicker. People are turning to nutritional therapies for two reasons:

- nutritional supplements provide healing and prevent disease;
- nutritional therapies are safe and do no harm.

The very illnesses and conditions found with greater frequency in children with Down Syndrome – bowel disorders, upper respiratory infections, heart disease, cancer and premature aging – are rapidly increasing in the general population. Diet and nutritional supplements such as vitamin E are routinely used to correct problems and prevent disease. Where Down Syndrome is concerned, however, parents are told that nutritional therapies are useless. Critics argue against vitamin therapy where Down Syndrome is present even if the problem is one helped by nutritional therapy in the general population.

And their reasoning makes no sense! If chronic bowel problems such as constipation or diarrhea are alleviated with supplementation of digestive enzymes, this remains true whether or not the bowel problem originates in Down Syndrome. In other words, we must treat the bowel problem, not the Down Syndrome. I strongly believe that it is unethical to withhold treatment that has proven beneficial AND safe for the same condition in the general population simply because the person has Down Syndrome.

The purpose of this book is to convey what's in between the extremes of something that is totally useless and something that will "fix" everything. I want parents to know where Nutri-Chem stands on safety and effectiveness. There is a host of evidence on individual nutrients needed in Down Syndrome and I want parents to have this ammunition to confront traditional doctors who are too often drug-oriented and not dealing with their children's needs. Parents need tools that will enable them to understand what works and what doesn't, what's truth and what's nonsense.

This book will provide you with information on health and illness, and the additional challenges posed by Down Syndrome. We'll look at how nutritional therapy can improve a child's quality of life both now and in the future. We'll examine studies that claim nutritional therapy is useless for children with Down Syndrome, and perhaps more importantly, we'll help you learn to assess research studies so you can decide for yourself what makes sense for your child. We'll also examine the implications of nutritional therapy for children with Autism.

## No cures. Just better health

What this book won't give you is a cure for Down Syndrome. That's not why Nutri-Chem provides laboratory testing and nutritional compounds. We're about "solving the problem" not solving the Down Syndrome. We want the same thing you want for your child: good health and all the benefits it can bring that enhance quality of life.

## Nutri-Chem today

From humble beginnings two decades ago, Nutri-Chem has developed into one vital part of an entity that our patients often refer to as "The Wellness Hospital." This "hospital" concept is comprised of three integrated entities:

(1) Nutri-Chem Pharmacy, a leading edge nutritional, pharmaceutical compounding pharmacy

(2) The International Center for Metabolic Testing (ICMT), a full blood and urine biochemical testing laboratory

(3) Metalife Biomedical Center, a complete medical center staffed by medical doctors, child psychiatrists and pharmacists.

Our professionals and staff working together in this integrated "Wellness Hospital" allows us to study on a child-by-child basis nutritional deficiencies in Down Syndrome and Autism. We have thoroughly explored these subjects and as a consequence of our research and approach, our practise has naturally grown to include other health issues. Some of these include extensive work in the areas of cancer, hormones, thyroid, brain wellness issues such as depression, ADD, pain management, other genetic biochemical disorders and many other "unknown" undiagnosed conditions that have stumped medical professionals. We have always used the approach of maximizing potential through laboratory testing and dietary and nutritional interventions on an individual basis. Of course as a pharmacist my approach also includes a thorough review of any pharmaceutical drugs patients have been prescribed which also has yielded many interesting results through the years!

We have dealt with tens of thousands of families in over 20 countries around the world. Our compounding and testing laboratories allow us to keep up-to-date not only with developments in Down Syndrome, but also with the most advanced nutritional science and testing procedures in the world. We have become a thriving practise serving the international Down Syndrome and Autism community.

Nutri-Chem is constantly re-evaluating nutritional therapies and testing procedures. Our team includes clinical biochemists, medical doctors, "child psychiatrists," homeopaths, nutritionists and pharmacists who collaborate to provide the most complete and effective approach to health improvement and disease prevention. We are always moving forward in our development as a comprehensive nutritional health organization.

# SECTION 1
# SETTING THE SCENE

## CHAPTER 1
### 20 Questions

## CHAPTER 2
### Understanding Vitamins

## CHAPTER 3
### Vitamins and Your Child's Intelligence

## CHAPTER 4
### Autism and Down Syndrome

# DANIEL'S STORY

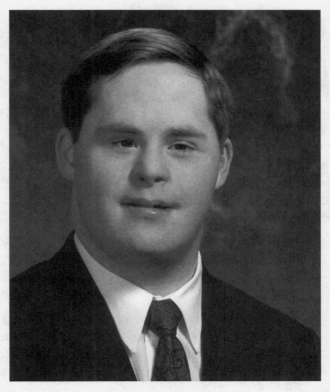

If Nutri-Chem created an award for its longest-standing MSB user, 22-year-old Daniel Pinsonneault would win. He started on the first MSB formula shortly after his first birthday, and he's been taking the nutritional supplement ever since. He'd also be a strong contender for an award of achievement: musician, computer operator, athlete, student council member, caregiver, and all-round number one son.

His mother, Eleanor, can't contain her pride in Daniel. "He has so many gifts. He loves music, and has started guitar lessons. He's wonderful helping people – I think that's where his real gifts are. He's very motivated, self-disciplined, and extremely responsible. He's such a wonderful son."

Eleanor's words are not just a mother's boast. At his recent work placement in an art studio specializing in working with people with disabilities, Daniel, who has Down Syndrome, earned high praise from his supervisor. His guitar teacher says he's seldom seen a student as motivated and disciplined as Daniel, and his high school classmates loved his sense of humour and caring attitude toward others.

When he attended his high school graduation, Daniel received a special Award of Achievement from Canada's Prime Minister. Eleanor calls it a "very, very sweet ending" to his school years.

Daniel completed a job placement where he helped run a unique art studio for people with disabilities. Daniel has spent the past three years at this same art studio where he did his first placement. The students do very original paintings and sculptures that hang in many public and private collections and the students receive a share of the proceeds. Presently they are doing a musical play. He's turning his athletic interests in swimming and basketball toward involvement in Special Olympics.

Currently, he's working in a rehabilitation hospital in a nearby city so he lives away from home during the week, and commutes on weekends. When he was home last weekend he said "Mom, I love my life!" What more can we wish for?

All this is pretty impressive for a young man who started life as a happy baby, but one who simply "wasn't thriving," Eleanor says. "When he was 11 months of age, he still could not roll over. He had serious digestive problems – if he ate peas, you'd see peas in his diaper." Eleanor sought out a local doctor who practiced holistic medicine and was well-known for her expertise in nutritional therapy and her work with children with special problems. The doctor had a long waiting list, but Eleanor persisted, writing letters and making phone calls until she finally got an appointment for Daniel. On the physician's advice, Eleanor started Daniel on Nutri-Chem's first MSB formula.

Eleanor recalls that Daniel's health started improving almost right away. "There was a change in his alertness. His digestion improved very quickly." Today, Eleanor acknowledges that it's hard to say that any one thing can be credited with her son's remarkable progress in life but feels certain that the long-term use of Nutri-Chem's MSB series was very instrumental in improving his cognitive abilities and physical well-being. "Daniel has had a loving family, a good diet, lots of fresh air. And people who have always prayed for him." Eleanor acknowledges that she believes "God was with this child."

# CHAPTER 1

# 20 QUESTIONS

WHEN THE TELEPHONE RINGS in my office at Nutri-Chem, I never know what awaits me on the other end of the line. Often over the years, the caller has been a mother or father of a child with Down Syndrome. Sometimes it's an expectant parent who has just learned that their baby will be born with this genetic disorder. Like all new parents, they're full of questions and anxieties. And like all parents who love their children, they start looking for ways to help their son or daughter overcome the challenges they know lie ahead. This search has led them to Nutri-Chem to find out whether nutritional supplements might benefit their child. Some know a great deal and challenge me with sophisticated questions and requests. Others are at the beginning of their odyssey of learning, and need very basic information.

**WHAT WILL I LEARN?**
- Will vitamins make my child smarter?
- Will vitamins improve my child's stature?
- Will vitamins improve my child's immune system?

Parents of children with Down Syndrome have been responsible for many of the positive social, medical, educational and legislative changes affecting the lives of their children that have occurred over the last 30 years. Life is better today for people with Down Syndrome – they are living longer, healthier lives and enjoying life in the community. Yet it's still true that in many areas of science, therapies proven effective for the general population are viewed with cynicism in the presence of that extra 21st chromosome.

As a pharmacist specializing in nutritional therapies, I have always been guided by one operating principle: solve the problem while doing no harm. When research validates a safe nutritional approach to a health problem, why withhold that therapy to a family simply because their child has Down Syndrome?

In my work, I see similar issues with regard to pain management. When someone is experiencing extreme pain, we compound and use transdermal analgesic pain killers for nerve pain, whether or not the pain has been caused by something genetic or by an accident. We are working on trying to solve the problem of pain regardless of the cause of that pain. Why is this approach not used in Down Syndrome? Why does the genetic component of Down Syndrome preclude a nutritional solution to problem solving even when that solution is proven helpful?

Information about specific problems and their links to nutrition can be found in the following chapters. But since so much of our work at Nutri-Chem has been driven by the problems parents bring to us, I'd like to give you brief answers here to some of the most commonly-asked questions I've had over the years. – K.M.

# Cause and research

### Is there anything I could have done before or during my pregnancy to prevent having a child with Down Syndrome?

New research is showing that two issues are implicated in the origin of the genetic disorder: functional folic acid deficiency, and oxidative stress in the mother during pregnancy. Folic acid is necessary for a process called methylation and formation of DNA. Oxidative stress damages cells and the genetic material they contain.

### What research has Nutri-Chem done in Down Syndrome?

As one example, Nutri-Chem enlisted the services of Dr. Marie Peeters-Ney to independently study the effects of MSBPlus on children with Down Syndrome. The study focussed on biological, developmental and immune issues before and after treatment with MSBPlus. Dr. Peeters-Ney's research concluded that the use of MSBPlus resulted in a 50% reduction of infections and a 65% increase in overall health of children with Down Syndrome.[1] We continue to undertake research in this area.

# Mental functioning (I.Q.)

### Will vitamins make my child smarter?

New studies show that vitamin supplementation has a positive impact on nonverbal I.Q. and that the effect is particularly dramatic in children who are malnourished (see *Chapter 3: Vitamins and Your Child's Intelligence*). Given the multiple effects of Down Syndrome on the body's ability to absorb, process and utilize nutrients, it is logical to believe that supplementation can have a positive effect on the I.Q. of children with Down Syndrome.

## Are there any drugs that will help my child's intelligence?

At this point there is no evidence that any drug improves intelligence in children. There are studies on piracetam and two small studies on aricept in Down Syndrome. Several small studies have shown benefits of piracetam in Down Syndrome. Other small studies have shown no benefits to piracetam in Down syndrome.[3, 4, 5, 6] Anecdotally, parents have reported significant benefits for children with Down Syndrome with the use of piracetam. At this point it would be difficult to say there is enough evidence in favour of or against the use of piracetam in Down Syndrome. Aricept has been used for treating patients with Alzheimer's disease to improve memory loss. It has shown small, if any, results and significant side effects.[7, 8]

# Appearance and speech

## Will vitamins change my child's stature?

Although it has not been studied long-term with children with Down Syndrome, we have evidence that chronic nutritional deficiencies will affect stature.[9, 10] Chronic zinc deficiency has been associated with short stature. Zinc supplements have significantly improved height and rate of growth in non-Down Syndrome children of short stature. Zinc's benefit on stature may be related to its positive effect on the thyroid. In Down Syndrome, both stature and thyroid problems are prevalent. It is important to make sure that a shorter heavier stature is not due to a nutritional cause rather than a genetic cause.

## My child is obese. What can I do?

The first thing to check is thyroid function. The problem with this test today is that the ranges of normal are becoming wider to catch more individuals with low thyroid function. So many lab tests are now showing low thyroid function that it is now deemed "normal."

In effect, we have moved the normal values to accommodate more people. This in turn means individuals are told they have normal thyroid function, even though they have all the symptoms of low thyroid including weight gain. Therefore, weight gain symptoms and basal metabolic rate through body temperature are simple ways to determine low thyroid function. Generally individuals with Down Syndrome have a lower metabolic rate which means they have reduced caloric requirements. However, wholesale restriction of food to combat obesity results in loss of muscle tone and significant nutritional deficiencies. The way to combat obesity is with the correct balance of fat, protein, low glycemic index carbohydrates and the correct fats and oils, together with nutritional supplementation.

### Will vitamins help my child's speech?

It has been proven that children with Down Syndrome who have fewer ear infections have better speech.[11] This can be accomplished by supporting your child's immune system with nutritional supplements. This is discussed in more depth in *Chapter 5: Understanding Antibiotics and Ear Infections*, and in *Chapter 9: The Immune and Thyroid Systems*.

## Immune system

### Will vitamins improve my child's immune system?

Yes, vitamins have been shown to improve the immune systems of children with Down Syndrome.[12, 13, 14, 15, 16] See *Chapter 9: The Immune and Thyroid Systems*.

### What can I do for my child's chronic sinus and respiratory infections?

Several nutrients are crucial to preventing infections by strengthening your child's immune system. These are known as the immune-boosters: vitamin A, zinc, vitamin C, echinacea and herbs that stimulate the immune system. At Nutri-Chem, we use a homeopathic product called Euphorbium. It is an anti-inflamatory that stimulates the body's immune and decongestant responses.

### What can I do about my child's skin problems?

Several key nutrients, namely vitamin A and zinc, have been shown to improve skin problems in children with Down Syndrome. Essential fatty acids such as EPA and DHA are also very effective in clearing up dry skin allergic response in children with Down Syndrome. Nutri-Chem compounds EPA, DHA, zinc and vitamin A in skin creams to accelerate the benefit of these nutrients.

## Digestion

### Are there any natural remedies to improve bowel function?

Absolutely. If your child is constipated, the first thing to check is thyroid function as the cause. The cornerstones of good bowel health are fibre, probiotics such as acidophilus, water, and good enzymes. If required, stool softeners can be used.

If your child has been on antibiotics, use lots and lots of acidophilus, a probiotic used to restore the healthy bacteria needed for healthy bowel movements. I often recommend upwards of 50 billion units of acidophilus a day for this purpose.

I also recommend Carbo Aid which contains enzymes that are found in the fragile and easily-destroyed lining of the bowel. Carbo Aid is especially helpful in reducing gas and bloating and any irritations that result from eating fruits, milks, starches and the acids found in vitamins. See *Chapter 7: The Digestive System* for more on this topic.

## Will vitamins help my teenager with Down Syndrome?

Individuals with Down Syndrome face different issues at different ages. Parents of young children are generally interested in maximizing growth and intellectual development. Parents of teenagers or young adults often have the same ongoing health concerns as well as issues associated with mood. Older adults with Down Syndrome face the issue of maintaining intellectual abilities. The answer is that certain symptoms and issues are more amenable to nutritional treatments during specific phases of growth and development. However, overall nutritional needs must be met at every stage: zinc is no less essential at 94 than it is at 4, though you don't have the same developmental issues at 94 that you have at 4. You are never too old to receive essential nutrients.

# Other medical issues

## What are the early signs of leukemia my child's doctor may not be aware of?

Children with Down Syndrome are at higher risk for leukemia. Early warning signs may include changes in the size and shape of red blood cells and specific changes in the Complete Blood Count (CBC) that may indicate early onset of certain leukemias. Your doctor should be made aware that there is a higher risk of leukemia in children with Down Syndrome.

## Are there lab tests that have proven beneficial for my child?

Absolutely. Even the most conservative physicians are recommending zinc assessments for children with Down Syndrome because it has been shown to be deficient.[17] Some of the lab tests I have found to be beneficial are: thyroid function tests, Complete Blood Count (CBC), iron, iron binding and

# DOWN SYNDROME

Down Syndrome was first identified by a British doctor, John Langdon Down, in 1866. Dr. Down described the set of common characteristics associated with the disorder, but it was not until 1959 that the cause of Down Syndrome was identified as being a third chromosome on the set of the 21st chromosome. This is the origin of the term "Trisomy 21" used to describe Down Syndrome.

Each cell in the body contains chromosomes which carry the genetic material DNA (deoxyribonucleic acid). As these cells, the basic unit of all living organisms, divide and form into different types (brain cells, liver cells, blood cells, etc.) the complete DNA is reproduced in each and every one. Thus, the extra chromosome found in Down Syndrome affects each and every process in the body.

Some of the problems associated with Down Syndrome have been well documented: small mouth and obstructed airways, heart defects, intestinal malformations, visual and hearing impairments and altered mental development. Children with

ferritin, as well as nutritional tests for antioxidants, amino acids, essential fatty acids, and organic acids which screen for a host of nutritional and biochemical abnormalities. The latter may include mythelation problems, heavy metal toxicity, copper deficiency, carnitine deficiency, B1 vitamin deficiency, biotin, B12 deficiency, lipoic acid and glutathion deficiency and mitocondrial defect.

## Are there any drugs that pose a risk to my child?

Yes. These include anaesthetics, methotrexate, anti-cholinergic drugs which may be used pre-operatively or for bladder or bowel disturbances, and certain antibiotics. (See *Chapter 6: Drugs and Down Syndrome* for further discussion on this topic.)

## My child is going to have surgery. Is there anything I should know that my doctor might not have told me?

Yes. Because of smaller airways, there is greater likelihood for airway obstruction. Children with Down Syndrome also have greater sensitivity to drugs, including pre-operative medications, and problems with drug clearance from their system.

### My child has Down Syndrome and Autism. Is there a link between these two conditions?

Absolutely. There is a much higher incidence of Autism in Down Syndrome. What is reported is that children with Down Syndrome are 20 times more likely to have Autism than children in the general population. Current opinion about Autism in the non-Down Syndrome population is that it is a genetic fragility which can be triggered by environmental effects or immunological disfunction.[18, 19] See *Chapter 4: Autism and Down Syndrome* for more.

### Are vaccines harmful for my child?

There is no proven link between vaccines and Autism. However, a recent Centre for Disease Control study linked thimerosal 9 mercury containing vaccines to neurological symptoms.[20] It is prudent at this point to ensure your child is using thimerosal-free or mercury-free vaccines.

# Vitamin safety

### Are vitamins harmful?

There is no evidence that in safe doses

Down Syndrome are at higher risk for thyroid problems, Autism and leukemia. They also have a universal susceptibility to Alzheimer's disease occurring at a young age.

The extra chromosome in Down Syndrome is like a factory worker on an assembly line who works twice as fast as the other workers. This will create too much of some materials, and not enough of others – the entire production process is affected.

There is still much to understand about the origins of Down Syndrome, and all the ways in which the presence of an extra chromosome affects the body's processes. In the meantime, great strides have been made toward improving the health and development for children now born with Down Syndrome. Medical services such as life-saving heart surgeries once denied to infants because they had Down Syndrome are now routinely performed. And access to schools, recreation and family life have resulted in developmental achievements previously thought impossible for people with Down Syndrome.

vitamins present any risk of harm. There are no reported deaths attributable to the use of supplemental vitamins. However, according to the U.S. Food and Drug Administration, there were 100,000 deaths in hospitals alone in one year caused by drug medications.[21]

## How do I know what brand of vitamins to take?

You should look at the quality assurance methods used by the compounding company. Are there regular assays (tests) of the product? Are there pharmaceutical chemists involved in the compounding? Does the company use top-quality ingredients? Is the taste made acceptable for your child without the use of unsafe chemical substances?

# Endnotes

1. Peeters, M., and MacLeod, K. (1999) Unpublished data. Reviewed in *Bridges* 4(1).

2. See endnotes on Chapter 3.

3. Vampirelli, P. (1978) [Piracetam in child neuropsychiatry. Clinical experimentation in a child neuropsychiatry department]. *Minerva Pediatrica.* 30(4): 373-6. Italian

4. Lobaugh, N.J. et al. (2001) "Piracetam therapy does not enhance cognitive functioning in children with down syndrome. *Archives of Pediatric and Adolescent Medicine.* 155(4): 442-8.

5. Kishnani, P.S., et al. (1999) "Cholinergic therapy for Down's syndrome." *The Lancet* 353: 1064-5.

6. Hemingway-Eltomey, J.M., Lerner, A.J. (1999) "Adverse effects of donepezil in treating Alzheimer's disease associated with Down's syndrome" (letter). *American Journal of Psychiatry* 156: 1470.

7. Birks, J.S. et al (2000) "Donepezil for mild and moderate Alzheimer's disease." *Cochrane Database Syst Rev.* (4): CD001190.

8. Rogers, S.L. et al. (1998) "Donepezil improves cognition and global function in Alzheimer disease: a 15-week, double-blind, placebo-controlled study." *Donepezil Study Group. Archives of Internal Medicine.* 158(9): 1021-31.

9. Perrone, L., et al. (1999) "Long-term zinc and iron supplementation in children of short stature: effect of growth and on trace element content in tissues." *Journal of Trace Elements in Medicine and Biology.* 13(1-2): 51-6.

10. Kaji, M., et al. (1998) "Studies to determine the usefulness of the zinc clearance test to diagnose marginal zinc deficiency and the effects of oral zinc supplementation for short children." *Journal of the American College of Nutrition.* 17(4): 388-91.

11. Whiteman, B., et al. (1986) "Relationship of otitis media and language impairment in adolescents with Down syndrome." *Mental Retardation* 24: 353-6.

12. Bjorksten, B., et al. (1980) "Zinc and immune function in Down's syndrome." *Acta Paediatrica Scand* 69: 183-187.

13. Fabris, N., et al. (1993) "Psychoendocrine – immune interactions in Down's syndrome: Role of zinc. In:" *Growth Hormone Treatment in Down's syndrome* (ed. S. Castells and K.E. Wisniewski, John Wiley & Sons Ltd, London) p203-217.

14. Franceschi, C., et al. (1988) "Oral zinc supplementation in Down's syndrome: restoration of thymic endocrine activity and of some immune defects." *Journal of Mental Deficiency Research* 32: 169-181.

15. Lockitch, G., et al. (1989) "Infection and immunity in Down syndrome: A trial of long-term low oral doses of zinc." *Journal of Pediatrics* 114: 781-7.

16. Anneren, G., et al. (1990) "Increase in serum concentrations of IgG2 and IgG4 by selenium supplementation in children with Down's syndrome." *Archives of Disease in Childhood* 65: 1353-1355.

17. Pueschel, S. (1999) "Gastrointestinal concerns and nutritional issues in persons with Down syndrome." *Down Syndrome Quarterly* 4(4): 1-11.

18. Kent, L., et al. (1999) "Comorbidity of autistic spectrum disorders in children with Down syndrome." *Developmental Medicine and Child Neurology* 41(3): 153-8

19. Kapell, D., et al. (1998) "Prevalence of chronic medical conditions in adults with mental retardation: comparison with the general population." *Mental Retardation.* 36(4): 269-79.

20. http://www.cdc.gov/nip/vacsafe/concerns/thimerosal/faqs-mercury.htm

21. Starfield, B. (2000) "Is US Health Really the Best in the World?" *Journal of the American Medical Association* 284(4): 483-85.

# MARIE EVE'S STORY

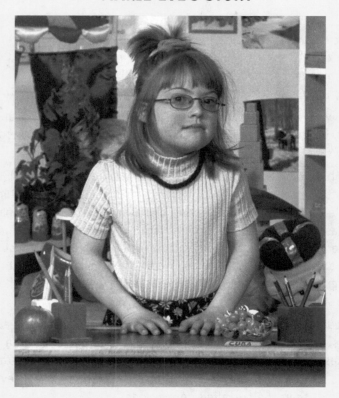

For Gerry Mulligan, vitamin therapies provide "answers, not miracles" for his daughter Marie Eve, who was a New Year's Eve gift when she was born nine years ago.

"When Marie Eve was born, her heart beat was very, very low," Gerry says. "Other than that, the only thing we noticed was that she was a little girl." With two grown sons, Gerry was delighted. The next day, doctors told Gerry and his wife, Luci, that Marie Eve likely had Down Syndrome. "We didn't know anything about Down Syndrome," he recalls. "We were a bit shaken, but Luci was great. She didn't see it as a problem, just something to cope with. For me it took a little time to feel the same way."

Gerry turned his engineer's mind to researching his daughter's genetic disorder. They started an infant stimulation program early, and Marie Eve's stamina improved dramatically. Her heart problem required surgery which she had successfully when she was a year-and-a-half old. It was around this time that Marie Eve started on Nutri-Chem's MSB formula.

"Kent MacLeod took a lot of time to explain and answer our questions. We felt it couldn't hurt her. It could not cure her Down Syndrome, but it made sense, so we decided to try it."

Marie Eve had severe bowel problems before she started on MSB. "She was very constipated. Within a very short time, less than a week, her bowel movements improved and she had more energy," Gerry says.

And if more proof was needed, two trips where Marie Eve's MSB was forgotten at home proved its benefits for his daughter. "Within a couple of days she started having bowel problems and constipation. The last time this happened was when we needed to go to Toronto for her ear problems and forgot to take her MSB. She was just miserable by the end of the two weeks we were there – tired, crying a lot, constipated and in pain. When we got back to her MSB, she got back to normal."

Although Marie Eve has some problems with her eyes, ears and joints, they don't hold her back much, Gerry says. She's in a Montessori primary school and her proud father says that not only is she seldom sick (only one mild cold this winter), she's "even healthier than the so-called normal kids."

Because of his proximity to Nutri-Chem's Ottawa location, Gerry visits often, reading "everything they have on health." He's preparing to start an early retirement from his job and looking forward to having extra time to spend with Marie Eve. "Improving Marie Eve's health changed our whole life. We exercise more, and have changed our diet to include such things as more fish. Health is not just a matter of taking a vitamin pill. "

# CHAPTER 2

# UNDERSTANDING VITAMINS AND MINERALS

*OFTEN WHEN PEOPLE TALK ABOUT VITAMINS, they also refer to the RDA or Recommended Dietary Allowance. What is the significance of this measurement? It's basically the level of nutrients the U.S. National Academy of Sciences determines is "judged to be adequate to meet the known nutrient needs of practically all healthy persons." When we look at nutritional supplements where deficiencies or illness exist, the RDA may not be sufficient. Nutri-Chem's MSB vitamin, mineral and amino acid formula incorporates the latest research on nutrition and Down Syndrome. Levels may vary but we are conscientious to ensure that levels that exceed RDA are without adverse effects and are completely safe. – K.M.*

## WHAT WILL I LEARN?

▸ There's more to health than simply the absence of disease.

▸ What vitamins and minerals do we need and why?

▸ Can food meet all of our nutritional needs?

▸ Do people with Down Syndrome have any special need for supplements?

# What is health?

Health is often defined as the absence of disease. But that's a little like defining happiness as the absence of sadness. Sure, if you're happy, that means you're not sad. But isn't happiness more than that? Happiness is about zest, energy, enjoyment.

So is health. Yes, if you're healthy, you don't have disease. But there's something more: you have the energy and vitality to engage in living, to learn new things, to connect with others in social relationships.

Adequate nutrition is essential to both warding off disease and promoting good health. Nutrients are the materials our bodies use for growth, energy and repair. Without them, our vital immune systems can't function, and our physical, mental and emotional abilities are impaired.

# What do we need and why?

When we're talking about nutrients, we're really talking about macronutrients (essential elements, water, carbohydrates, proteins and fats) and micronutrients (vitamins, minerals, essential fatty acids and amino acids). A healthy body requires a mix of all nutrients present because they don't work in isolation. It's like a house that needs a foundation, walls, connecting doors, roof, furnace and chimney. Every part is dependent on the existence of the others. With nutrients, some are catalysts (activators) or co-factors for others. For example, vitamin E and zinc are required for proper vitamin A metabolism; riboflavin (vitamin B2) is needed for vitamin B6; vitamin D is required for calcium absorption. Many vitamins and minerals act as coenzymes, enabling enzymes (the workers of life) to perform their functions in growth, energy and healing. As we look at specific nutrients and their roles, it's important to remember the law of nutritional synergy. A healthy body requires a mix of all nutrients present because they do not work in isolation.

A cautionary note: The following descriptions should be read as capsule comments only – the role and interaction of nutrients is more complex than can be included in such a summary.

## VITAMINS

These nutritional materials cannot be made by the body; they must be obtained from food or supplements. They are divided between fat-soluble which can be stored in the body, and water-soluble which pass from the body within a few days and cannot be stored.

### DEFINING MOMENT

**Enzymes and coenzymes:** An enzyme is a protein that helps chemical reactions work. A coenzyme is a molecule (like a vitamin or mineral) that helps the enzyme work better.

**WATER-SOLUBLE VITAMINS:**

- **VITAMIN B1** (Thiamine): water soluble, essential for energy metabolism
- **VITAMIN B2** (Riboflavin): water soluble, essential for energy production by cells, antibody production, vision, metabolism
- **VITAMIN B3** (Niacin): water soluble, needed for circulation, metabolism, digestion
- **VITAMIN B5** (Pantothenic Acid): water soluble, aids in formation of antibodies and conversion of nutrients into energy, needed for gastro-intestinal system and formation of neurotransmitters
- **VITAMIN B6\*** (Pyridoxine): water soluble, essential for most body functions including brain, nervous system, red blood cell production, immune system
- **VITAMIN B12\*** (Cyanocobalamin, Methylcobalamin, Hydroxycobalamin): water soluble, prevention of anemia, aids folic acid for red blood cells, needed for digestion and absorption, important for cellular formation and health, prevents nerve damage

- **FOLIC ACID\***: water soluble, essential for brain function, energy and red blood cell formation, strengthens immune system white blood cells, acts as coenzyme in DNA and RNA synthesis for cell division and reproduction, important in pregnancy for normal fetal development
- **BIOTIN**: water soluble, needed for metabolism and aids in cell growth
- **VITAMIN C** (Ascorbic Acid): an antioxidant, important for tissues, hormone formation and metabolism
  - \* Folic acid, and vitamins B6 and B12 and certain amino acids are essential for proper functioning of the SAM cycle (S-adenosyl-methionine). Please refer to *Chapter 12: One Mother's Story* for more information.

## Fat-soluble vitamins:
- **VITAMIN A** (Retinol): fat soluble, essential for the immune system, also vision, skin and mucous membranes
- **VITAMIN D** (calciferol): fat soluble, needed for absorption of calcium, needed for regulation of calcium and phosphorus metabolism, important for healthy bones
- **VITAMIN E** (tocopherol): antioxidant, protects cell membranes, vitamin A and fats from oxidative stress/free radicals
- **VITAMIN K** (menaquinone/phylloquinone): fat soluble, needed for blood clotting, healthy bones, liver.

In addition to these vitamins, carotenoids and coenzyme Q10 are important to note. There are more than 600 identified carotenoids, a class of compounds which give fruits and vegetables their colour (orange, yellow and red). More and more health benefits of these compounds are being discovered each year. The most widely studied carotenoid is beta-carotene, which your body converts to vitamin A. Coenzymes are molecules that are necessary as catalysts for enzymes. Coenzyme Q10 is very important for energy production. Protein, carbohydrates and fats provide energy for our body. But before our cells can use this energy, it has to be converted to a usable form. Coenzyme Q10 has an essential role in helping the energy from food be converted to a usable form for our cells.

## MINERALS

These nutrients are essential for all cell function and structure. Plants and plant-eating animals get minerals from soil and water, and we in turn obtain minerals from eating these plants and animals, or by taking supplements. Our bodies need some minerals in large quantities (calcium, chloride, magnesium, phosphorus, potassium, sodium and sulfur) and others called trace elements in smaller amounts. This doesn't mean, however, that the lower levels required indicate they're of lesser importance to our bodies. All minerals are essential.

### MACROMINERALS:

- **CALCIUM**: vital for bones and teeth, also in heart health and muscles
- **CHLORIDE**: regulates water balance; part of hydrochloric acid, found in stomach, which is necessary for proper digestion
- **MAGNESIUM**: necessary for energy production, nerve function, needed for calcium and potassium absorption and essential for muscle relaxation and function and neurotransmitter regulation
- **PHOSPHORUS**: bones and teeth, important in genetic material
- **POTASSIUM**: nervous system and heart, cells, blood pressure
- **SODIUM**: regulates water balance
- **SULFUR**: stabilizes proteins (in skin, hair, nails), part of insulin

**TRACE MINERALS:**

- **CHROMIUM**: energy (glucose metabolism)
- **COPPER**: functions in red blood cell and collagen formation, role in energy, healing and neurotransmitter regulation
- **FLUORIDE**: important for bones and teeth
- **IODINE**: important for healthy thyroid functioning
- **IRON**: essential for blood cells and and muscle tissue, immune system and formation of neurotransmitters and healthy bowel lining
- **MANGANESE**: metabolism, nerves, immune system, proper blood sugar, joint functioning
- **MOLYBDENUM**: nitrogen metabolism, cell function
- **SELENIUM**: antioxidant, works with vitamin E, important for heart, recycles glutathion
- **ZINC**: essential for immune system and brain function, role in protein synthesis and collagen formation, blood sugar control, key component in over 200 enzymes essential for life.

# Can food supply everything we need?

In a perfect world, yes, food can provide adequate nutrition to maintain health for most people. The first problem with this statement, however, is that we don't live in a "perfect" world. In our world, foods are grown in soil depleted of mineral content, artificially ripened after early harvesting to meet the needs of long-distance markets, and laden with cancer-causing pesticide chemicals. The result? Foods that are practically devoid of nutritional value.

Here's just one example: zinc, a nutrient deficient in children with Down Syndrome and one that is important for brain and immune function, does not appear in plants until late in their growth cycle. Modern fertilization methods speed up growth, producing plants with virtually no zinc content. Without crop rotation, the soil itself is lacking zinc.

Today, it's virtually impossible to get the nutrients we need from our diet. In reality, half of children don't eat even one fruit or vegetable daily. In the U.S., only 26% of children, ages 2-19 years, eat the recommended 5 or more servings of fruits and vegetables a day. Children eat only 3.4 servings of fruits and vegetables a day; a small increase from 3.1 servings in 1991.[1] It's even worse in Canada: only 20% of Canadian children eat the recommended 5 daily servings of fruit and vegetables. For 50% of children, their sole source of daily vegetable is french fries.[2]

In my experience, supported by the research, this poor diet is amplified in children with Down Syndrome due to difficulties in feeding and eating, and problems with taste and sensation of food. Yet parents whose children will eat only french fries are told by medical professionals that all their children's nutritional requirements are supplied in their food – they don't need to supplement with vitamins and minerals.

Only after talking to hundreds of parents did I realize the great difficulty they were having trying to insist that their child with Down Syndrome or Autism eat nutritional foods. Most of these parents were approaching a state of desperation in just trying to get their child to eat anything, let alone any of the recommended food groups!

There's also the "exaggeration factor" – the fact that when asked by a doctor or nutritionist, on average people exaggerate their nutritional intake. When I am doing consultations with patients, they often say they consume twice as much calcium or drink half as much coffee as they actually do. It's connected to being in a position where some authority will judge our worthiness. For people with children, it's rooted in fear that they'll be perceived as bad parents. Doctors tell people to "eat a well-balanced diet," never asking what the person is actually eating on a daily basis to determine nutritional deficiencies.

We also need to look at what we mean by "health." Instead of seeing this merely as an absence of disease at a given moment in time, we need to view health as a continually-evolving state. Some of the most serious illnesses and life-threatening diseases can be in their infancy in our bodies, growing and taking hold without our knowledge until symptoms rear their ugly head. Thus, we need to consider the disease-prevention requirements of our bodies where nutrition is concerned – not just how much of a certain substance we need for our health today. Finally, we need to look at the additional nutritional requirements arising from specific problems associated with Down Syndrome.

## Supplements and Down Syndrome

Many essential nutrients have been proven to be low in children with Down Syndrome. These include vitamins A, C, E, folate, zinc, selenium, iron and essential fatty acids. Of these, low levels of antioxidant nutrients are of particular concern because of the role they play in the immune system. (See *Chapter 9: The Immune and Thyroid Systems* for more on this.) Without a strong and healthy immune system, your child is sicker more often, more likely to be prescribed antibiotics which disrupt bowel function and nutrient absorption, and is more susceptible to life-threatening diseases in the future.

For instance, children with Down Syndrome may have a functional deficiency of folate.[3, 4] The RDA intake may be adequate for people without Down Syndrome, but if that third chromosome has affected processes in the body so that it is not processing folate in the normal manner, the recommended intake may not be sufficient, and then a functional deficiency may result.

When researchers have studied the diets of children with Down Syndrome, they have found that the recommended intakes of several nutrients are not adequate. One study showed that for children with Down Syndrome under the age of 6, 42% consumed less than two-thirds of the requirement for iron; 30% consumed less than two-thirds of the RDA for vitamin C.

The diets of children aged 5 to 11 are more complete, although half of the children did not meet 80% of the RDA for vitamin E, calcium and zinc.[5, 6]

Inadequate levels of zinc, selenium, vitamin A, and vitamin E are found in the blood of children with Down Syndrome.[7, 8, 9, 10, 11]

It is recommended that all children with Down Syndrome be tested for zinc and selenium levels.[12]

Antioxidants and certain essential fatty acids also play a crucial role in the brain. (See *Chapter 10: The Brain* for more on this.) This is important for brain function and has long-term implications, especially in Down Syndrome where we see higher rates of Alzheimer's disease and the presence of its characteristics at an early age.

Cystathionine-beta synthase (CBS) is an enzyme found on the 21st chromosome. Its activity is elevated in Down Syndrome. This affects the SAM cycle (S-adenosyl-methionine), which in turn affects folate levels and methylation reactions. Methylation reactions are important for normal metabolism, and the formation of DNA, hormones, and many other molecules (See *Chapter 12: One Mother's Story* for more on this).

Supplements in the right combinations and correct dosage can supply nutrients missing or impossible to get from food. They also supply nutrients which your body is supposed to manufacture on its own, but can't because essential cofactors are lacking.

Are nutrients deficient in children with Down Syndrome because of the genetic order? And if so, what mechanisms are at work? These are questions researchers continue to study. In the meantime, children with Down Syndrome display altered levels of nutrients and high rates of the illnesses and disease that result. Parents, rightfully, want help for their children regardless of whether or not the problems are rooted in Down Syndrome.

## Closing comments from Kent:

*I was contacted by a mother asking about nutritional supplements for her child with Down Syndrome. She said she believed in good nutrition and also in using supplements. In fact, she told me, her family all took supplements including herself, her husband, and their three other children – with one exception. She did not give supplements to her child with Down Syndrome. "Why not?" I asked. "Because our doctor said they aren't proven to raise I.Q. in Down Syndrome," she replied. "Is the rest of the family taking supplements for I.Q.?" I asked. Of course the answer was no. They were taking nutritional supplements to keep healthy in mind and body, and to prevent disease. This is the very reason to give supplements to a child with Down Syndrome. – K.M.*

# Endnotes:

1. 1994 U.S.D.A. data on fruit and vegetable consumption

2. *Heart and Stroke Foundation Report Card on Health*, 1998

3. Wachtel, T.J.; Pueschel, S.M. (1991) "Macrocytosis in Down syndrome." *American Journal of Mental Retardation* 1991 Jan;95(4): 417-20

4. David, O., et al. (1996) "Hematological studies in children with Down syndrome." *Pediatric Hematology and Oncology* 1996 May-Jun;13(3):.271-5

5. Luke, A., et al. (1996) "Nutrient intake and obesity in prepubescent children with Down syndrome." *Journal of the American Dietetic Association* 96: 1262-67.

6. Calvert, S., et al. (1976) "Dietary adequacy, feeding practices, and eating behavior of children with Down's syndrome." *Journal of the American Dietetic Association* 69: 152-156.

7. Franceschi, C., et al. (1988) "Oral zinc supplementation in Down's syndrome: restoration of thymic endocrine activity and of some immune defects." *Journal of Mental Deficiency Research* 32: 169-181.

8. Kadrabova, J., et al. (1996) "Changed serum trace element profile in Down's syndrome." *Biological Trace Element Research* 54: 201-206.

9. Lockitch, G., et al. (1989) "Infection and immunity in Down syndrome: A trial of long-term low oral doses of zinc." *J Pediatr* 114: 781-7.

10. Shah, S., et al. (1989) "Antioxidant vitamin (A and E) status of down's syndrome subjects." *Nutrition Research* 9: 709-15.

11. Neve, J., et al. (1983) "Selenium, zinc and copper in Down's syndrome (trisomy 21): blood levels and relations with glutathione peroxidase and superoxide dismutase." *Clinica Chimica Acta* 133: 209-14.

12. Pueschel, S. (1999) "Gastrointestinal concerns and nutritional issues in persons with Down syndrome." *Down Syndrome Quarterly* 4(4): 1-11

# JONATHAN'S STORY

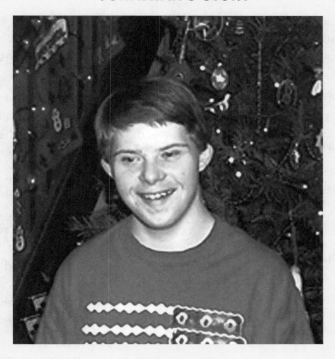

At 18, Jonathan Hale is an accomplished and engaging young man. He's responsible for household chores including all the laundry in his family of four, has held a part-time job at his high school where he does well in his studies, and has a large CD collection that reflects his wide taste in music – everything from opera to rap. But it's his good health and cheerful personality that his mother Natalie credits to Nutri-Chem's MSB formula which Jonathan has been taking for more than five years.

"Before starting on MSBPlus, Jonathan always had some type of infection even though I'd always had him on various vitamin supplements," says Natalie. "After he started taking MSB, the infections were just gone. It got to the point where he was the only one in the family who never got a cold."

It isn't only Jonathan's physical health, however, that has benefitted from his Nutri-Chem formula. In addition to having Down Syndrome, Jonathan was diagnosed with severe Attention Deficit Hyperactivity Disorder (ADHD) and Oppositional Defiant Disorder (ODD) which his mother describes as being "way past stubborn." It meant extreme difficulty at home and at school and Natalie sought out all kinds of natural remedies after disastrous results from prescribed drugs such as Ritalin and anti-depressants.

Then five years ago Natalie was speaking with a Nutri-Chem chemist who explained how the brain functions differently in Down Syndrome and about supplements that can prove beneficial.

## What is DMAE?

DMAE (Dimethylaminoethanol) is a chemical naturally produced in the human brain. It is thought to be used by the body in converting choline to the neurotransmitter acetylcholine. DMAE increases the concentration of choline in the bloodstream because it enhances the rate at which free choline enters the bloodstream from other tissue. DMAE increases the levels of choline in the brain due to its superior ability to cross the blood-brain barrier.

Acetylcholine, which is essential for brain function, has been proven low in Down Syndrome. DMAE studies show DMAE increases alertness, improves behaviour and mental function in children with Down Syndrome, and improves learning and memory.

Jonathan started taking the DMAE Combination (Dimethylaminoethanol, vitamin B12, L-methionine, Folic Acid and Acetyol-L-carnitine). There were no results for the first six months, Natalie recalls, until the dosage was increased to what turned out to be the right amount. (Jonathan doesn't have individualized testing because he refuses to let anyone administer a needle to him.)

"We were staying in a closeknit summer community at that time, where everyone knows each other. Literally overnight after we got the DMAE formula quantity correct, Jonathan changed. The feedback from everyone in the community was immediate. 'What happened to Jonathan?,' they all said. 'He's like a different person.'"

No longer a reclusive, unfriendly boy, Jonathan started smiling, engaging with people, behaving cooperatively. Since then, he hasn't looked back. His mother emphasizes the "HUGE!!!" difference in his cheerfulness at school. He follows instructions with minimal prompts, has warm and friendly relations with others, and is "just a different kid who does very well socially," says Natalie with pride.

# CHAPTER 3

# VITAMINS AND YOUR CHILD'S INTELLIGENCE

*IN ALL OF MY YEARS WORKING IN THIS FIELD, I have been struck by how what I hear from parents, and what I read in studies, is at odds. Parents tell me, again and again, how much their child has improved once nutritional supplementation is in place. Yet there were 4 studies of I.Q. in Down Syndrome in the early 80's where I.Q. was shown not to be affected by supplements. It is these studies which have formed the basis for the notion that nutrients do not affect I.Q. in Down Syndrome. Now when these studies are dissected piece by piece to see what they really prove you will note that there are limitations and bias in these studies. (You'll find more about both of these areas in Appendix A: Existing Studies and their Limitations.) Then, literally as I was completing writing this book, a study was brought to my attention that helped the pieces fall into place. Turns out that the lack of study support for the benefits of nutritional supplementation on intelligence hinges on one fundamental issue: we've been studying the wrong kind of intelligence. – K.M.*

**WHAT WILL I LEARN?**

▸ How the kind of intelligence being measured makes all the difference

▸ The nonverbal intelligence connection

▸ How parents often see what researchers miss

# What I.Q. tests really test

I.Q., or intelligence quotient, sounds like such a scientific term, one that should be easy to determine, like measuring your height or your weight: you're 5 foot, 7 inches tall; you weigh 160 pounds; your I.Q. is 110. But it's not really that simple. How you score on an I.Q. test depends on the test's design. This becomes especially critical when trying to test the I.Q. of someone whose literacy skills are limited. (It's also an issue when testing people of different cultures or social classes. I.Q. test questions can be subtly biased against people of lower incomes, for instance.) In an effort to measure I.Q. in those with limited literacy skills, researchers have typically resorted to testing verbal intelligence. But even verbal intelligence tests fail to measure changes in the most basic form of intelligence: nonverbal intelligence.

**DEFINING MOMENT**

**Non-verbal intelligence**
Non-verbal intelligence measures how the brain organizes and processes information as opposed to verbal intelligence which looks at the words and understanding of words.

There are many problems with the existing studies on nutritional supplementation and I.Q. (as you'll see in *Appendix A*). But one of the most fundamental issues is that these tests have not tried to measure nonverbal intelligence. When it comes to children who have deficits at the most basic levels of intellect, failing to measure nonverbal intelligence is a bit like a mechanic pronouncing that the car he's working on is fine – without checking to see if there's any gas in the tank. Another example of the problems with verbal intelligence would be illustrated in a situation where a group of kids are given an I.Q. test in Spanish. The kids that speak Spanish will score a higher value on this verbal I.Q. test. This measure of intelligence rests on a person's knowledge of Spanish words and how well they can communicate. This knowledge (or intelligence) relates to many environmental (where I was born and raised) and socialization issues rather than to intelligence issues (i.e. how I can organize and process information in my brain). This group of kids' ability to speak and understand the words in Spanish is not going to be affected by any supplements they take, but rather will be impacted by their home and social environment. Whereas if you look at non verbal intelligence and note that a child's brain is better organized then you can draw your own conclusions as to the measure of a child's intelligence.

## The Schoenthaler Analysis

That's where the Schoenthaler study comes in. This study looked at the effects of low-dose multivitamin and mineral supplementation in improving the intelligence of children and young adults. The study reviewed 13 randomized, double-blind trials (which, as you know, are the gold standard of research trials). These studies involved almost 1,500 children aged 6 to 17 in 15 public schools in Arizona, California, Missouri, Oklahoma, Belgium, England, Scotland and Wales, as well as 276 young adult males aged 18 to 25 in two American correctional facilities. All of the studies use standardized tests of nonverbal intelligence (the Wechsler Intelligence Scale for Children-Revised, the Wechsler Adult Intelligence Scale or the Calvert Non-Verbal Test).

What did the study find? The group taking vitamins in each study performed better on average than the placebo (also known as the control) group in nonverbal I.Q. regardless of formula, location, age, race, gender or research team composition. The probability of 13 randomly selected experimental groups always performing better than 13 randomly selected control groups is 1/2 to the 13th power – or about 1 in 10,000. It's safe to say this didn't happen by accident: something is going on here that is causing the experimental groups to perform better. That something was low-dose multivitamins and minerals.

The mean difference across all of the studies was 3.2 I.Q. points. That doesn't sound like a lot, does it? But what the studies also found was that in the experimental groups, the standard deviation in I.Q. points was consistently larger in the experimental groups than in the control groups. What this means is that a few children in each study were producing large differences, rather than each child experiencing a 3.2 point gain.

The studies found that not all children responded to supplementation. But the children who experienced the larger point gains were those who were low in micronutrients to begin with. It makes perfect sense: like cars without enough gas, children without enough micronutrients showed the most dramatic benefits when supplemented.

The studies also showed something that the parents I work with have been telling me all along: the first noticeable improvement in these children was psychological. That is, they demonstrated better mood, better memory, better attention and better eye-hand coordination. These are all the kinds of things that parents and teachers tend to notice, and that researchers testing verbal I.Q. would miss.

What supplements were common to the vitamins that reported positive results? Zinc, iron, manganese, B-vitamins, vitamin A, vitamin D and vitamin E were linked to the positive outcomes. As well, iron was noted in one study to be particularly associated with improving nonverbal intelligence in those test subjects who had poor iron status as judged by low ferritin.

## What does this mean for all children?

In the U.S., The Healthy Foundation is so convinced that vitamin supplementation will make a difference in the lives of children that it has undertaken a program to supply free multivitamins to at-risk children. This program is supported with funding from Congress, as well as from corporations and private donors. Find out more about Vitamin Relief USA, Operation I.Q. and The Healthy Foundation at www.healthfound.org.

## What does this mean for children with Down Syndrome?

The children in the studies examined by Schoenthaler did not have Down Syndrome. Does that mean that these results don't apply to children with Down Syndrome?

Of course not. If multivitamin supplementation has a positive effect on children who don't have Down Syndrome, why would it not also have a positive effect on children with Down Syndrome? And most importantly, the children who showed the biggest gains were those who had the biggest vitamin and mineral deficits to begin with. As you'll see in later chapters, there are numerous physiological reasons that cause children with Down Syndrome to experience vitamin and mineral deficits even when they are eating a healthy diet.

So what should a parent do? Research proves that children with Down Syndrome have physiological problems that interfere with their body's ability to utilize the vitamins and minerals found in a normal diet. There is no evidence to show that multivitamin and mineral supplementation is harmful to your child. There is good – and growing – evidence that supplementation will produce positive and sometimes dramatic results in children. The answer is clear. At worst, supplementation will not harm your child. At best, it could result in dramatic improvement.

## Closing comments from Kent:

*I've had parents tell me again and again that their child's doctor is opposed to multivitamin supplementation because "there's no proof it does any good." In fact the proof is so strong – and the risk of harm so low – that I believe doctors should be challenged to prove to parents why they shouldn't supplement. – K.M.*

# Endnotes

1. Benton, D. "Micro-nutrient supplementation and the intelligence of children." *Neurosci Biobehav* Rev 2001 Jun;25(4): 297-309.

2. Benton, D. *Vitamin and mineral intake and human behaviour.* In: Smith, Andrew P. (Ed);

3. Jones, Dylan M. (Ed). (1992). *Handbook of human performance, Vol. 1: The physical environment; Vol. 2: Health and performance; Vol. 3: State and trait.* (pp. 25-47). San Diego, CA, U.S.: Academic Press, Inc. 1117 pp. ISBN 0-12-650354-0.

4. Benton, David. "Vitamin/mineral supplementation and the intelligence of children: A review." *Journal of Orthomolecular Medicine.* Vol 7(1) 1992, 31-38.

5. Benton, D., Buts, J.P. "Vitamin/mineral supplementation and intelligence." *Lancet* 1990 May 12; 335 (8698): 1158-60 Comment on: *Lancet.* 1990 Mar 31; 335 (8692): 744-7.

6. Publication Types: "Clinical trial. Comment Controlled clinical trial." Letter. Comment in: *Lancet.* 1990 Jul 21; 336 (8708): 175-6

7. Benton, David, Cook, Richard "Vitamin and mineral supplements improve the intelligence scores and concentration of six-year-old children." *Personality & Individual Differences.* Vol 12(11), 1991, 1151-1158.

8. Benton, D., Roberts, G. "Effect of vitamin and mineral supplementation on intelligence of a sample of schoolchildren." *Lancet.* 1988 Jan 23; 1(8578): 140-3

9. Boggs, Unabelle R., Scheaf, Allen, Santoro, David, Ritzman, Robert "The effect of nutrient supplements on the biological and psychological characteristics of low IQ, preschool children." *Journal of Orthomolecular Psychiatry.* Vol 14(2), 1985, 97-127.

10. Boivin, M.J., Giordani, B. "Improvements in cognitive performance for schoolchildren in Zaire, Africa, following an iron supplement and treatment for intestinal parasites." *J-Pediatr-Psychol.* 1993 Apr; 18(2): 249-64.

11. Carlton, R.M., Ente, G., Blum, L., Heyman, N., Davis, W., Ambrosino, S. "Rational dosages of nutrients have a prolonged effect on learning disabilities." *Altern Ther Health Med* 2000 May; 6 (3): 85-91

12. Carroll, H.C.M. "A psychometric critique of Nelson et al.'s 1990 paper: Nutrient intakes, vitamin-mineral supplementation and intelligence in British schoolchildren." *Personality & Individual Differences.* Vol 18(5), May 1995, 669-675.

13. Crombie, I.K., Todman, J., McNeill, G., Florey, C.D., Menzies, I., Kennedy, R.A."Effect of vitamin and mineral supplementation on verbal and non-verbal reasoning of schoolchildren." *Lancet.* 1990 Mar 31; 335(8692): 744-7 Comment in: *Lancet.* 1990 May 12; 335(8698): 1158-60

14. Crombie, I.K., Todman, J., McNeill, G., Florey, C.D. "Vitamin/mineral supplementation and intelligence." *Lancet* 1990 Jul 21; 336(8708): 175-6 Comment on: *Lancet*. 1990 May 12; 335(8698): 1158-60

15. Emery, P.W. "Vitamin/mineral supplementation and non-verbal intelligence." *Lancet* 1988 Feb 20; 1(8582): 407-9.

16. Eysenck, Hans J. "Raising I.Q. through vitamin and mineral supplementation: An introduction." *Personality & Individual Differences*. Vol 12(4), England: Elsevier Science Ltd. 1991, 329-333.

17. Eysenck, Hans J., Schoenthaler, S. J. "Raising IQ level by vitamin and mineral supplementation." In: Sternberg, Robert J. (Ed); Grigorenko, Elena L. (Ed). (1997).

18. *Intelligence, heredity, and environment*. (pp. 363-392). New York, NY, US; New York, NY, US: Cambridge University Press; xvii, 608 pp. ISBN 0-521-46489-7.

19. Grantham McGregor, S.M., Walker, S.P., Chang, S.M., Powell, C.A. "Effects of early childhood supplementation with and without stimulation on later development in stunted Jamaican children." *Am-J-Clin-Nutr*. 1997 Aug; 66(2): 247-53.

20. Lozoff, B., Jimenez, E., Wolf, A.W. "Long-term developmental outcome of infants with iron deficiency." *N-Engl-J-Med*. 1991 Sep 5; 325(10): 687-94.

21. Naismith, D.J., Nelson, M., Burley, V.J., Gatenby, S.J. "Can children's intelligence be increased by vitamin and mineral supplements?" *Lancet* 1988 Aug 6; 2(8606): 335.

22. Nelson, M. "Vitamin and mineral supplementation and academic performance in schoolchildren." *Proc Nutr Soc* 1992 Dec; 51(3): 303-13

23. Nelson, M., Naismith, D.J., Burley, V., Gatenby, S., Geddes, N. "Nutrient intakes, vitamin-mineral supplementation, and intelligence in British schoolchildren." *Br J Nutr* 1990 Jul; 64(1): 13-22

24. O'Dea, J., Rawstorne, P. "Consumption of dietary supplements and energy drinks by schoolchildren." *Medical Journal of Australia* 2000 Oct 2; 173(7): 389.

25. Pagliari, H. Claudia. "Effects of nutritional supplements on intelligence: Comment on Schoenthaler et al.'s paper." *Personality & Individual Differences*. Vol 14(3), Mar. 1993, 493.

26. Pollitt, E. "Iron deficiency and educational deficiency." *Nutrition-reviews*. Apr 1997. v. 55(4) p. 133-141.

27. Peritz, E. "The Turlock vitamin-mineral supplementation trial: a statistical reanalysis." *J Biosoc Sci* 1994 Apr; 26(2): 155-64

28. Pollitt, E., Gorman, K.S., Engle, P.L., Rivera, J.A., Martorell, R. "Nutrition in early life and the fulfillment of intellectual potential." *J-Nutr*. 1995 Apr; 125 (4 Suppl): 1111S-1118S 1995

29. Pollitt, E., Watkins, W.E., Husaini, M.A. "Three-month nutritional supplementation in Indonesian infants and toddlers benefits memory function 8 y later." *Am-J-Clin-Nutr.* 1997 Dec; 66(6): 1357-63 1997.

30. Ricciuti, Henry N. "Nutrition and mental development." *Current Directions in Psychological Science.* Vol 2(2) Apr 1993, 43-46.

31. Rippere, V., Benton, D. "Vitamins, minerals and IQ." *Lancet* 1988 Sep 24;2 (8613): 744-5.

32. Roberts, G. "Boost your child's brain power: how to use good nutrition to ensure success at school." *Wellingborough: Thorsons,* 1988. 142pp. ISBN: 0-7225-1752-1 Wellingborough:

33. *Thorsons,* 1988. 142pp. ISBN: 0-7225-1752-1.

34. Schoenthaler, S. J. "Effects of nutritional supplements on intelligence: Comment on Schoenthaler et al.'s paper: Response." *Personality & Individual Differences.* Vol 14(3), Mar 1993, 493.

35. Schoenthaler, Stephen J., Amos, Stephen P., Doraz, Walter E., Kelly, Mary A., et al. "Controlled trial of vitamin-mineral supplementation on intelligence and brain function." *Personality & Individual Differences.* Vol 12(4), 1991, 343-350.

36. Schoenthaler, Stephen J., Amos, Stephen P., Eysenck, Hans J., Peritz, E., et al. "Controlled trial of vitamin-mineral supplementation: Effects on intelligence and performance." *Personality & Individual Differences.* Vol 12(4), 1991, 351-362.

37. Schoenthaler, S.J., Bier, I.D., Young, K., Nichols, D., Jansenns, S. "The effect of vitamin-mineral supplementation on the intelligence of American schoolchildren: a randomized, double-blind placebo-controlled trial." *Journal of Alternative & Complementary Medicine* 2000 Feb;,6(1):,19-29.

38. Schoenthaler, S.J., Bier, I.D. "Vitamin-mineral intake and intelligence: a macrolevel analysis of randomized controlled trials." *J Altern Complement Med* 1999 Apr;5 (2): 125-34

39. Schuitemaker, G.E. "Nutrition and behaviour." *Journal of Orthomolecular Medicine.* Vol 3(2), American Assoc. of Orthomolecular Medicine. 1988, 57-60.

40 .Sigman, Marian, Whaley, Shannon E. "The role of nutrition in the development of intelligence." In: Neisser, Ulric (Ed). (1998). *The rising curve: Long-term gains in IQ and related measures.* (pp. 155-182). Washington, DC, US: American Psychological Association. xv, 415 pp. ISBN 1-55798-503-0 (hardcover)

41. Singh, Mahendra P, Agrawal, Padma "Effect of nutrition on intellectual development." *Perspectives in Psychological Researches.* Vol 10(2), Oct , 1987, 25-29.

42. Smith, W.B. "Commentary on Schoenthaler et al: vitamin and mineral supplements – is the methodology sufficient to support the conclusions?" *J Altern Complement Med* 2000

43. Snowden, Wendy "Evidence from an analysis of 2000 errors and omissions made in IQ tests by a small sample of schoolchildren, undergoing vitamin and

**Chapter 3: Vitamins and Your Child's Intelligence**

mineral supplementation, that speed of processing is an important factor in IQ performance." *Personality & Individual Differences*. Vol 22(1), Jan. 1997, 131-134.

44. Southon, S., Wright, A.J., Finglas, P.M., Bailey, A.L., Loughridge, J.M., Walker, A.D. "Dietary intake and micronutrient status of adolescents: effect of vitamin and trace element supplementation on indices of status and performance in tests of verbal and non-verbal intelligence." *Br J Nutr* 1994 Jun; 71(6): 897-918.

45. Soewondo, S. "The effect of iron deficiency and mental stimulation on Indonesian children's cognitive performance and development." *Kobe-J-Med-Sci.* 1995 Apr; 41(1-2): 1-17.

46. Swensson, Marjorie. "Nutrition and Its Effects on Learning." 43p.; *M.S. Practicum*, Nova University. 1990

47. Todman, John, Crombie, Iain, Elder, Leona. "An individual difference test of the effect of vitamin supplementation on non-verbal IQ." *Personality & Individual Differences*. Vol 12(12), 1991, 1333-1337.

48. U.S. Congress 102nd. *Meeting the Goals: Collaborating for Youth. Hearing Before the Committee on Labor and Human Resources, United States Senate. One Hundred Second Congress, First Session. On Examining the Need To Provide Comprehensive Services To Youth To Help the Nation Meet the Education Goals of School Readiness, Dropout Prevention, Improved School Achievement, and Drug and Violence Free Schools and To Examine What the Federal Government Can Do To Support and Expand Social Service Programs for Youth.* U.S. Government Printing Office, Superintendent of Documents, Congressional Sales Office, Washington, DC 20402. 1991

49. van den Briel T., West, C.E., Bleichrodt, N., van de Vijver, F.J., Ategbo, E.A., Hautvast, J.G. "Improved iodine status is associated with improved mental performance of schoolchildren in Benin." *Am J Clin Nutr* 2000 Nov;72(5): 1179-85

50. "Vitamin claims challenged". *Times* 1988 Aug 12.

51. "Vitamin/mineral supplementation and non-verbal intelligence." *Lancet* 1988 Feb 20;1 (8582): 407-9

52. Walker, S.P., Grantham Mcgregor, S.M., Powell, C.A., Chang, S.M. "Effects of growth restriction in early childhood on growth, IQ, and cognition at age 11 to 12 years and the benefits of nutritional supplementation and psychosocial stimulation." *J-Pediatr.* 2000 Jul; 137(1): 36-41 2000.

53. Weissberg, Roger P., Gullota, Thomas P., Hampton, Robert L., Ryan, Bruce A., Adams, Gerald R. "Enhancing Children's Wellness." *Healthy Children 2010. Issues in Children's and Families' Lives, Volume 8.* The John & Kelly Hartman Series. Sage Publications Inc., 2455 Teller Road, Thousand Oaks, CA 91320. 1997

54. Yudkin, John "Intelligence of children and vitamin-mineral supplements: The DRF study: Discussion, conclusion and consequences." *Personality & Individual Differences.* Vol 12(4), 1991, 363-365.

# JORDAN'S STORY

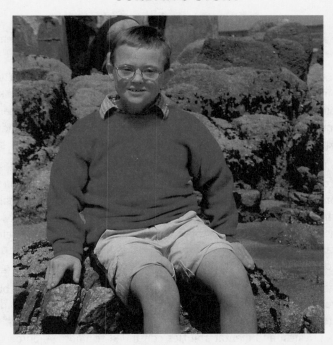

Jordan Blevins, now 8, started on Nutri-Chem's MSB formula in the midst of a crisis. Within just over a year, he'd gone from a happy, healthy six-month-old to a boy who was sick with a high fever every single day, was throwing up undigested food 30 to 40 times a day, had round-the-clock croup, almost no bowel movements and continuous mucous secretions from his nose and eyes. His breath had a foul odour, and his urine smell was so bad, his mother Linda says, "even the dogs left the room."

But what horrified Linda most was that Jordan had stopped growing. "He had gone from the fiftieth percentile on the growth chart, to six standard deviations off the chart. I had bells and whistles going off in my head that something was wrong, but I had total blind faith in the medical system that they had my child's best interests at heart. When I asked how come my son was sick all the time, throwing up all the time, I was told this was normal for kids with Down Syndrome."

As Linda sought answers to her son's problems, she learned about nutritional deficiencies and metabolic changes in children with Down Syndrome. In defiance of medical and advocacy groups who told her "you will kill your child if you put him on vitamins," Linda started Jordan on a regime of growth hormone, zinc, cod liver oil, and vitamin C. She saw improvements – Jordan's mucous cleared up, he was more alert, he started growing. Massage treatments helped him have bowel movements.

"Part of my awakening was the realization that you can't have poop sitting in your system because it goes putrid." Her efforts weren't supported by Jordan's doctors who were, Linda says, "absolutely no help. It was okay with them that he was constipated and refluxing 30 to 40 times a day."

"Kent MacLeod at Nutri-Chem was one of the first people who said that yes, there was something we could do for Jordan. At first, I was just calling Kent for advice and purchasing vitamins at a local health food store. But as I learned more about nutritional deficiencies and metabolic changes in Down Syndrome, I felt Kent's experience with other children like Jordan was valuable, so I started using MSB."

In addition to nutritional supplements, growth hormone and elimination of lactose in Jordan's diet, the Blevins were working on a neurological rehab program at the National Academy of Child Development in Salt Lake City, Utah. By 18 months of age, Jordan went from what his mother calls "zero development" to a vocabulary of 20 words and reading flash cards. He was walking at 19 months and climbing stairs soon after.

For some time, Linda had suspected that Jordan's vaccinations were to blame for his earlier problems. Each time he had received immunization shots, Jordan's health had suffered. At 21 months of age, he had another round of vaccinations and while his physical and mental abilities continued to improve, Jordan's behaviour began exhibiting signs of Autism. He developed acute auditory sensitivity – a lawnmower three blocks away put him into a state of extreme anxiety, flipping his hands in front of his eyes all the while. He became obsessive about lining up objects and spinning wheels. He lost his vocabulary, by then at 100 words, and the ability to recognize colours and shapes. Worst of all, he lost his ability to focus and interact with others.

As Linda looked for answers, she became convinced that dangerously high levels of neuro-toxic mercury in Jordan's immune vaccinations were to blame for her son's deteriorating condition. She learned of the link between Autism and Down Syndrome, rooted in metabolic disturbances, and had a biochemical profile done of Jordan. Out of 10 essential amino acids, her son was low in 8. "I sent the results to Kent MacLeod and he made recommendations on how we could change his MSB formula.

Now 8 years old, Jordan has had no further vaccinations. He has remained on MSB and growth hormones, and Linda has removed glutin and caseine from his diet. He still has some Autistic behaviours such as minor vocalizing and arm movements when he's excited. "If you created a scale where zero represents no Autism, and 100 extreme Autism, Jordan would be a 25," says Linda. "He is learning to read and school tests put him in the low range of a normal I.Q. He is back on the regular growth charts, and is actively engaged in sports. I believe we turned him around with nutritional therapy. Vitamins are not a cure-all, but if you can keep a kid healthy and growing, then something's going right."

# CHAPTER 4

# AUTISM AND DOWN SYNDROME

OVER THE LAST 20 YEARS, I've spoken to thousands of parents of children with Down Syndrome. Of these, some stand out in my mind. These are parents whose children display the core characteristics pointing to a diagnosis of Autism, but who have never been diagnosed as such by medical professionals who view the problems as related to their Down Syndrome. These are teenagers who have never spoken a word, or children who are extremely socially withdrawn (a trait uncharacteristic of Down Syndrome). Some perform repetitive, meaningless actions which they cannot control. Despite all this, only rarely has one of these parents told me their child has been diagnosed with Autism spectrum disorder (ASD). And even then, the dual diagnosis has almost always been made first by the parents themselves.

## WHAT WILL I LEARN?

- Whether children with Down Syndrome are at greater risk for Autism
- Why early diagnosis matters
- How to improve your child's outcome in cases of Autism
- The link between Autism and heavy metal exposure

Through my work in recent years with the ICMT biomedical laboratory and with many Autism groups, and now through our Metalife Biomedical Center, it is obvious that Autism in Down Syndrome is grossly under-diagnosed. The purpose of this chapter is to raise awareness and provide some insight into a variety of biological treatments that have proven effective in Autism.

## How common is it?

*Reported incidence of Autism in Down Syndrome is approximately 10% according to Howlin, Wing and Gould[1] while others estimate it to be as low as 1%[2]. Such variations are due to disagreement about diagnostic criteria and incomplete documentation of cases over the years. Parents report that medical doctors attribute autistic behaviours in their children to their Down Syndrome despite evidence to the contrary. Dr. Bernie Rimland has noted to me that there is a parent group for children who are diagnosed as both Autistic and Down Syndrome: Info Centre for Dual Diagnosis: Downs and Autism, 3124 Henneberry Road, Jamesville New York, 13078; telephone 315-677-3844. Dr. George Capone at Kennedy Kreiger has written an excellent overview of current knowledge of Down Syndrome and ASD. Capone states his belief that the true incidence of Autism in Down Syndrome is between 5 and 7%, a rate 20 times higher than in the general population[3] This points to a link between genetic or other factors and the incidence of Autism, a point covered in more detail later in this chapter. – K.M.*

# Does gender matter?

In a word, yes. Dr. Capone's review of the literature on this subject dating back to 1979 indicates that gender is a grossly neglected issue where Autism is concerned. He reviewed 36 reports on Down Syndrome and ASD. Of the 31 cases included that cited gender, 28 were males and only 3 female.[4] While we don't yet know the cause of Autism and any link to Down Syndrome, the gender issue emerges again in a British study on brain development and the effect of nutritional supplements on subsequent I.Q. In this study (examined in more detail in *Appendix A*), boys had three times the benefit from supplements in terms of subsequent I.Q. This showed that, in general, brain development in boys was more sensitive to nutritional factors than that of girls. This finding concerning gender has been relatively ignored for its potential impact on Down Syndrome and ASD.

Fatty acids essential to brain development are also associated with gender. Males have a higher fatty acid requirement than females, so deficiencies create greater problems in the developing male brain. It is noteworthy in this context that Attention Deficit Disorder (ADD) and Attention Deficit Hyperactivity Syndrome (ADHS) have a higher incidence among males.

## Autism among the non-Down Syndrome population

A good description of Autism is a "genetic fragility" colliding with nutritional and environmental factors. That is, some people are born with a genetic predisposition to Autism, which is then triggered by nutritional and/or environmental factors. The incidence of Autism in the non-Down Syndrome population has increased dramatically during the last 20 years. This is not attributable to any change in the genetic makeup of the population. Instead, we must look to environmental and nutritional factors for this increase in Autism in the general population. It is important to note Dr. Capone's observation that children with congenital heart disease, anatomical gastro-intestinal problems, neurological disorders (seizures, dysfunctional swallowing, severe hypotonia or diminished muscle tone, and motor delay) and opthamologic problems were all more likely to have ASD. Clearly links to these conditions and to environmental factors must be studied further where Autism is concerned.

## What should I look for?

In an article commenting on the Howlin, Wing and Gould study, Dr. Robert Pary[5] notes that the following characteristics were found in four boys (ages 8, 9 and two age 11) who had both Down Syndrome and Autism:

- impaired social interactions as evidenced by: lack of awareness of others' feelings, inability to seek comfort, impaired imitation, lack of social play and poor peer relationships;

- impaired communication including poor eye contact and nonverbal communication, impaired imagination and stereotyped speech;

- stereotyped routines including motor movements, preoccupation with parts of objects, distress over trivial changes, insistence on routines and preoccupation with a narrow interest in something.

Two of the four boys disliked physical contact and all were aggressive to peers. All four children flapped their arms and three of the boys rocked back and forth. Some of their fixated interests included fitting things into boxes, watching certain videos, spinning things and flickering candles and switches. They were attached to certain objects (leaves, sticks, a pink hairbrush, a piece of hosepipe) and all had fixed daily patterns and/or places for objects.

Dr. Pary notes that while Autism is typically diagnosed by school age in the non-Down Syndrome population, the diagnosis is often made much later in children with Down Syndrome. The Howlin et al study indicates that parents reported difficulty getting professionals to consider Autism in their children as the reason they were falling behind in school.

In my experience with parents of non-Down Syndrome Autistic children, most become very concerned about their children by the age of two and almost universally a diagnosis of Autism is made before the children start school. In contrast, I cannot recall a single child with Down Syndrome whose diagnosis of Autism has occurred before the age of four. More typically I consult with parents whose children are in their teens or much later and who have autistic characteristics, yet I am the first person to broach the issue of Autism with them. Clearly, the medical profession has a problem diagnosing Autism in Down Syndrome.

It is important that early diagnosis take place so that children with a dual diagnosis can benefit from specialized treatments and appropriate educational and behavioural interventions. Dr. Capone is a leading expert in this area, and I encourage parents to read his work.

## The drug approval issue

Physicians commonly tell parents that biological treatments such as nutrients and vitamins are not "approved" for Autism. What parents need to realize, however, is that while certain drugs may be tried for alleviating symptoms of Autism, no drug is so-called "approved" for treatment of ASD. Despite this fact, Nutri-Chem clients report that their children are prescribed any number of drugs including psycho-active drugs (those affecting the brain) for treatment of Autism. None of these drugs are "approved" for such treatment and when analyzed, some are found to have been prescribed to counteract side effects of other drugs the child is taking.

One of the best resources for parent research is the Web site of the Autism Research Institute (www.Autismresearchinstitute.com). Dr. Bernie Rimland of the Institute has tracked thousands of cases of parents of Autistic children with respect to their use of a variety of drugs (both prescription and non) and nutrients including benefits and side effects of each. NONE of the substances under review are "approved" in the treatment of Autism, and the Institute recognizes that there is no benefit in giving a non-approved prescription drug over a non-approved nutritional supplement. The database included on the Web site is important because it reports benefits and adverse events for all substances.

There is now a large number of medical practitioners affiliated with the Autism Research Institute who have come to be known as DAN (Defeat Autism Now) practitioners. They recognize the "genetic baggage" that comes with a label of Down Syndrome, and how it limits the diagnosis and treatment of Autism.

As a practising pharmacist, I am constantly amazed by the high number of medical practitioners who regularly use unapproved, risky drug therapies on young children while attacking the use of safe, rational complementary therapies on the grounds that they are "unapproved." I am also appalled at the discrimination parents of children with Down Syndrome must face in seeking a diagnosis of Autism and appropriate treatment. Routinely such parents are accused of being "in denial" because they are looking for improvements in their children's Autistic symptoms. If parents seek biomedical alternative solutions to their children's Autism-related behavioural problems, they are ostracized for not accepting their children because of their Down Syndrome!

## Treatment for a child with Down Syndrome and Autism

Nutri-Chem has worked with many parents of children with a dual diagnosis. From this experience, and drawing on the work of DAN practitioners, we recommend that parents consider the following treatments as proposed by Dr. Sidney Baker.[6]

### Applied behaviour analysis

This is a specific type of training for children with learning problems that has proved beneficial and warrants investigation by parents for use with their autistic children.

### Dietary modification

Parents consistently report that removal of casein (the main protein in milk and dairy products) and gluten have proven beneficial for their children. To accurately assess whether or not a child has improved, it is recommended that all casein be removed for a period of three weeks, and all gluten for a minimum of three months.

**CASEIN:** Children with Down Syndrome have a higher incidence of lactose (the sugar found in milk) intolerance. This results in gas, bloating or diarrhea. Casein, which is extremely hard to digest, differs from lactose. Evidence of a morphine-like compound (casomorphine) has been found in ASD children caused by improper handling of casein.[7, 8, 9] By measuring casomorphine in urine, we are able to recommend a casein-free diet which has proved to have a positive effect in these children. In following a casein-free diet, it is important to supplement calcium particularly because children with Down Syndrome have a higher incidence of bone loss.

**GLUTEN, CELIAC DISEASE AND GLIADORPHIM:** As noted in a later chapter on digestion, children with Down Syndrome have a much higher incidence of celiac disease than the general population. Celiac disease is a specific immune system response to gluten in the diet. How it may be related to Autism is under study. Norwegian researcher Dr. Karl Reichelt has suggested that in children with Autism, a neuro-toxic compound is made from gluten called gliadorphim.[10, 11] It is obvious then that children with celiac disease and/or Autism will benefit from complete removal of gluten. Tests such as IGG food reactions or gliadorphim may be helpful for parents in choosing a course of action. However, many parents have reported benefits simply by removing gluten from their child's diet even when test results have been negative or inconclusive.

**PROTEIN:** Studies of children with ASD have consistently identified involvement of at least two systems: 1) dopamine which regulates movement, posture, attention and reward behaviours; and 2) serotonin which regulates mood, sleep and feeding behaviour. Clinically, drugs which modulate serotonin and dopamine have been used to treat ASD, sometimes with success. The *American Journal of Clinical Nutrition* reported a study where serotonin was significantly elevated in the brain using whey protein.[12, 13] Serotonin comes from tryptophan, a dietary amino acid which is a constituent of proteins. Dopamine comes from tyrosine which is also a dietary constituent of protein.

One of the dietary modifications Nutri-Chem clients have found beneficial is to improve and regulate protein intake. Most kids are generally protein-malnourished and children with gastro-intestinal problems have additional deficiencies caused by diets that are restricted by choice or design. It is beneficial to supplement their diet with egg white protein, pea protein or a customized amino acid protein to meet the basic protein requirements of approximately one-half gram per pound of body weight per day (for example, a 60-pound child needs 30 grams of protein each day as a minimum). Balancing this protein throughout the day may have further benefits on behaviour. For our 60-pound example, the 30 grams of protein could be split into three ten-gram servings. Logical Choice Whey Protein is of particular benefit in children who do not have a milk sensitivity. It is predigested, easy on the gut, and has additional immune enhancers and regulating peptides that cause rapid flooding of the brain with these amino acids. The good news is that results of protein supplementation are often rapid and significant.

**GASTRO-INTESTINAL ISSUES:** Gastro-intestinal problems are more common in children with Down Syndrome and Autism. Obvious signs include constipation, diarrhea, gas, bloating and reflux reactions. DAN (Defeat Autism Now) practitioners and parents have noted significant benefits to children with Autism by improving their bowel function and digestive systems. Both Autism-specific therapies (see below) and general digestive aids may prove beneficial. The latter includes acidophilus in high doses (we recommend Nutridophilus Innoculator), Carbo Aid and general enzymes for the prevention of constipation including stool softeners, lactulose, magnesium or a combination of these.

**SPECIFIC BOWEL SUPPORT AGENTS IN ASD:** Enzymes made by Klaire Laboratories (which makes the enzyme Seranaid), Kirkman Laboratories (which makes the enzyme Enzynmaid) and Houston Nutraceuticals are among those suggested for cleanup of undigested substances specific to Autism. DAN practitioners have also reported significant benefit from antifungal therapy. Tests to detect the presence of fungus include blood (antibodies to yeast), urine (yeast metabolites identified), and stool (fungus either cultured or identified under the microscope). It should be noted, however, that the response to antifungal therapy as stated by Dr. Sidney Baker and other DAN practitioners is not dependent on these lab tests. Stated another way, a child with test indicators may have little or no benefit from antifungal therapy and conversely, a child who shows nothing on tests for fungus may have dramatic improvement.

Parents shouldn't overlook nature's own fungus suppressor – healthy bacteria. Often, fungus flourishes because antibiotics, preservatives and other toxins have wiped out this healthy flora, and this opens the door to opportunists such as fungus that are antibiotic-resistant (see *Chapter 5* for more on the important topic of antibiotics). In an unhealthy environment this fungus grows like the mold on an orange skin and is tough to get rid of. Sufficient levels of natural antifungus (three pounds in a healthy adult) will choke out this fungus. However, in extreme cases drug therapy is needed. One of the safest of these is Nystatin which is not absorbed into the body but is virtually 100% eliminated in the feces. Nystatin does have the short-term effect of worsening symptoms of the fungus problem. This happens because of the high amount of what is called the kill-off reaction – the death and dying-off of the fungus byproducts that are not being absorbed back into the body. However, in the longer term, children experience favourable outcomes from this treatment.

Systemic drugs (those absorbed into the body) such as Nizerol, Diflucan or Sporinox can be used as well as antifungal therapy. Results can be positive from these where Nystatin has failed. Adverse effects from these drugs can occur although this is rare.

Over-the-counter products with antifungal properties are s.boulardii, caprylic acid, olive leaf extract and garlic, among others.

## Nutrition in Autism

Surveys at the Autism Research Institute show that nutritional supplementation has consistently shown significant benefits for kids with Autism.[14] These general formulas are essentially multivitamins with significantly raised levels of B6 (many times more than the Recommended Daily Allowance or RDA) and magnesium at levels approximating the RDA. Other nutrients play a crucial role as well. One of these is zinc. Low levels of zinc in Down Syndrome have far-reaching consequences for virtually every system in the body. Researchers are now looking at its role in Autism.

Studies have shown that the copper zinc ratio is 40% higher in Down Syndrome than in a control group.[15] Dr. William Walsh at the Pfeiffer Treatment Center has found abnormal levels of copper and zinc in blood studies of 503 non-Down Syndrome Autistic patients.[16] He postulates that this abnormality (which is believed to be genetic) results in impaired brain development and extreme sensitivity to toxic metal and other environmental substances. This disorder is often unnoticed in infancy and early childhood until aggravated by a serious environmental insult.

There are two key proteins that regulate zinc and copper. They are metallothionein (14 amino acids with a high proportion of cysteine) and carnosine. In humans, metalothynine proteins regulate the blood levels of zinc and copper, detoxify mercury and other heavy metals and assist in neuronal development. Research indicates that the body's metallothionein needs zinc with adequate cysteine and glutathione. In Down Syndrome, there are low levels of glutathione and zinc which can be expected to deplete metallothionein.

Metallothionein has a role as an antioxidant as well. Children with Down Syndrome have greater oxidative stress which depletes all levels of the antioxidant proteins such as glutathione and metallothionein, vitamins E, A and C, and minerals such as selenium. Enhanced oxidative stress can cause significant damage to the adult brain (such as Alzheimer's disease). It is conceivable that this enhanced oxidative stress may be a causal factor in Autism in Down Syndrome. In addition to conservative recommendations for zinc testing, it is desirable to test for antioxidant nutrients.

Carnosine is a dipeptide consisting of two amino acids: beta-alanine and histadine. It has a role in the brain in regulating copper and zinc and has a detoxifying function for aldehydes which have been shown to be a factor in Alzheimer's disease. A disturbance of copper-zinc ratios would affect carnosine which is copper-zinc sensitive. Use of carnosine in seizure disorders associated with Autism is currently being studied.

Vitamin A levels in Down Syndrome have been shown to be depressed. In children with Down Syndrome, it is relatively common to have a child turn "orange" (hypercarotenemia) from excess betacarotene in the body that cannot be converted to active vitamin A. Once again, zinc enters the picture as it is essential to normal levels of active vitamin A. Dr. Mary Megson and parents report improvements in their autistic children with the use of cod liver oil supplements containing vitamin A and essential fatty acids essential for the structure and function of the brain.[17] In particular, omega-3 fatty acid (ecosopentanoic acid), demonstrated to be low in both Alzheimer's and Down Syndrome, has been shown to significantly improve mood in depression and function in schizophrenia. Dr. Patty Kane reports improvements of function in autistic children by improving fatty acid levels.[18]

**SAM AND FOLIC ACID:** In *Chapter 8*, we will outline the crucial role played by the SAM cycle and folic acid. Disturbances in this cycle and folic acid deficiency are related to genetic defects such as neurotube defects, colorectal and some other cancers and some types of leukemia. Here are a few points of importance:

- Folic acid is not in an active form, it must be converted in the body to folinic acid (methylenetetrahydrofolic acid or THF).

- As many as 30% of mothers of children with Down Syndrome have been found to have an abnormality in the enzyme that forms folinic acid.[19]

- Disturbances in this pathway are found in celiac disease, leukemia, rheumatoid arthritis and schizophrenia.[20]

- Relatives of autistic individuals have high rates of psychiatric disorders.[21]

- Not everyone can transform folic acid into active folinic acid but only folic acid is measured in routine blood tests.

Misconceptions about folic acid can have tragic consequences as evidenced in a case report of a young girl who died of folinic acid deficiency despite showing normal total serum folic acid in a routine blood test.[22] The extent of this problem is just beginning to be investigated.

In Down Syndrome, we know that the SAM cycle is adversely affected. We know that methylation problems can be associated with psychiatric disorders. It makes sense to undertake complete folate cycle testing and studies including folinic acid to understand the impact of the SAM cycle disorders on Autism and Down Syndrome.

At Nutri-Chem, we recommend that children with a dual diagnosis of Down Syndrome and Autism be supplemented with biologically active folinic acid. This is because:

- folinic acid is very safe,
- we do not currently have widespread ability or education regarding testing for folic acid cycle defects, and
- if we wait for medical doctors to recommend this supplementation, it will take decades.

This is evidenced by the fact that it took doctors 20 years to recommend folic acid supplements to women of child-bearing age after it had been shown in the early 1980's to prevent neural tube defects. Dr. Rimland has noted that the first paper he was aware of, linking folic acid deficiency to neural tube defects is Hibbard, E.D., Smithells, R.W. "Folic acid metabolism and human embryopath," *Lancet* 1965-1, page 1254. Dr. Rimland goes on to say that "this work was ignored for about 20 years until several large-scale studies were done confirming it, in the early 80's and after another dozen or so years the medical establishment finally got around to recommending that pregnant women take folic acid supplements!"

## Heavy metals

Heavy metals cause damage by competing with essential minerals such as iron, zinc and copper. In addition, heavy metals bind with sulph-hydryl groups in proteins, rendering them ineffective. Interference in critical paths (as in the Kreb's cycle noted below in the section on testing) can be disastrous. Heavy metals deplete glutathione because it is sacrificed in the removal of these toxins. It is important to improve levels of glutathione and selenium which is essential for the recycling of glutathione.

The connection between heavy metals is much discussed, highly controversial and generally misunderstood. The main reason for the misunderstanding is the similarity shown between Autism and heavy metal toxicity in both lab findings and symptoms. Medical doctors make several mistaken assumptions where heavy metals (arsenic, mercury, lead and cadmium) are concerned.

**DIFFERENT REACTIONS:** The first of these mistaken assumptions is that the same dose of mercury will cause the same health problems in all individuals regardless of genetic, environmental or nutritional status. An identical dose of mercury given to 30 children will result in some dying and some having no symptoms at all. In between these two extremes, a number of systems can be affected: behaviour, bowel and brain (both short and long term). Add in certain variables such as low iron levels and mercury toxicity can increase by as much as tenfold.

**WHAT TESTS REVEAL:** The second mistaken assumption relates to blood tests and their ability to detect heavy metal toxicity. A blood test for heavy metals will only detect recent exposure. Yet heavy metals are buried deep in tissues with a half-life of as long as 27 years in the case of mercury.[23] More reliable testing involves "provoking" the release of these heavy metals using chelating agents, then collecting a sample over a number of hours. For this process the drug DMSA is administered under physician supervision and urine is collected over the next four to six hours. This is important because DMSA is actually a treatment, and starts to remove the deep-seated mercury and other heavy metals. Urine organic acid testing is extremely sensitive to observing the toxic effects of heavy metals on the essential flow of electrons through this energy cycle. When heavy metals are present, elevations of intermediates start to occur. (*Note:* Some practitioners treat patients for heavy metals before receiving direct evidence of toxicity based on their experience of its benefit without safety concerns.)

**DEGREE OF TOXICITY:** The third wrong assumption about heavy metals is that they are all equally toxic. Current evidence suggests that while all heavy metals are toxic, mercury is capable of causing significant damage in amounts much lower than previously thought. The only proven safe level is none at all. Where Alzheimer's disease is concerned, work at the University of Calgary suggests that if there is a toxic element involved, mercury is the culprit.[24]

**WHO BENEFITS FROM REMOVAL:** The fourth incorrect assumption about heavy metals is that the only people who benefit from their removal are those with low blood metal levels. Not so. This is because heavy metals stress a whole variety of systems in the body – some we can measure, and some we cannot. These are set out below.

Systems we can measure include the following:

- Iron status via a complete iron panel. Iron deficiency increases heavy metal toxicity.
- Zinc testing. Zinc deficiency increases heavy metal toxicity.
- Kreb's cycle intermediates and interference. This will assist in determining cofactors such as B vitamins, glutathione and lipoic acid. Kreb's cycle is a series of metabolic reactions that helps to convert the energy in food into a useable form for our cells.
- Antioxidant testing. Coenzyme Q10 deficiency will exaggerate heavy metal toxicity. Heavy metals increase oxidative stress. Vitamin C decreases lead levels, as much as 50%.
- Glutathione status. Levels are fundamental to Down Syndrome, Autism and heavy metals.

Systems we cannot measure include the following:

- Bowel function. Most mercury is excreted in the feces. If a child is constipated, it is important to address by heavy metal removal.
- Genetics. Even within the Down Syndrome group, individual genetics increase susceptibility to Autism. Interestingly, susceptibility to Alzheimer's disease is

genetically different in the Down Syndrome population. In the non-Down Syndrome population the likelihood of getting Alzheimer's is high when a gene is present that is highly sensitive to mercury. We can measure this genetic type but until we create the program to prevent heavy metal attack, we don't really have an approved therapy for prevention of Autism or Alzheimer's.

**HEAVY METAL REMOVAL PROGRAM:** Information about a Heavy Metal Removal Program can be found on Web site of the Autism Research Institute (www.autismresearchinstitute.com). It includes a consensus statement by DAN practitioners associated with the Institute.

At Nutri-Chem, our recommendation with regard to heavy metal removal is to follow the Autism Research Institute protocol. In addition, we emphasize the following:

- protein in the diet through nutritional counselling and amino acid testing;
- adequate antioxidant status evidence by blood and urine testing basic blood work, Complete Blood Count (CBC), liver and kidney function and ferritin, iron and iron binding capacity testing;
- folinic acid and methyl B12 supplementation;
- essential fatty acid testing;
- complete support of bowel function (see above on gastro-intestinal issues);
- glutathione support that includes selenium, glutathione and cysteine.

This complete biochemical and nutritional support should be given for 11 consecutive days followed by three days of a prescribed chelator (binds to heavy metals for removal) according to the Autism Research Institute protocol.

# Secretin

Secretin is a hormone that works on the pancreas to stimulate release of sodium bicarbonate into the small intestine. Its benefit for children with Autism was thought to be related to their prevalent gastro-intestinal bowel problems.[25] Recent studies have shown no such benefit.[26, 27, 28] Evidence is now emerging that while children with bowel disturbances can't respond to secretin, it does improve brain function in autistic kids with healthy bowels. No side effects of secretin supplement have been recorded. The issue of secretin and its controversy illustrates the many challenges with introducing new concepts to medicine. I have included Dr. Bernie Rimland's editorial "Secretin update: a negative placebo effect?" which illustrates the many challenges facing the medical approach to new therapies.

## Closing comments from Kent:

*Autism is 20 times more prevalent in children with Down Syndrome as compared to the regular population. Furthermore, this number is likely to be dramatically under-reported. Parents of children with Down Syndrome must be aware of the risk factors for Autism and seek a diagnosis where symptoms warrant so that appropriate interventions can be undertaken. Underlying issues that increase the risk for Autism include low glutathione or antioxidant status, zinc depletion, gastro-intestinal disturbances with higher rates of celiac disease, methylation problems via SAM cycle disturbance and medical and genetic problems with unknown origin. The value of testing can't be underestimated as early warning signals for this debilitating disease. – K.M.*

# Secretin update: a negative placebo effect?

Bernard Rimland, Ph.D.
Autism Research Institute
4182 Adams Avenue
San Diego, CA 92116

The placebo effect is a consistent tendency for patients to over-report benefits from a treatment that they believe in. To control for placebo effects, researchers conduct blind or double-blind experiments, in which the subjects do not know whether they are being given an active treatment, e.g., a drug, or a placebo. The double-blind study is considered to be the "gold standard." But the gold is tarnished.

Blind studies are employed because patients are human beings, and as such have expectations of either help or harm from the treatments they are subjected to. But the experimenters are also human beings, and they too have expectations, which it would be unwise to overlook. The researchers' expectations may have strong and perhaps overriding effects on the results of the experiments they conduct. That is our concern here.

Recently there have been accounts in the popular media, as well as in the professional literature, of trials of the use of the hormone secretin. On the one hand we have many reports of dramatically good results attested to by the parents of autistic children and by their physicians. Children who have never slept the night through begin to sleep soundly, immediately after the secretin infusions. Children who have had chronic diarrhea for months or years suddenly begin having normal bowel movements. Children who have never spoken, or made eye contact with their parents, suddenly begin to show remarkable improvement in these symptoms. Very convincing!

However, the half dozen or so research studies which have been formally reported have (supposedly) not produced positive results. Why these conflicting conclusions?

Skeptics have repeatedly tried to explain away the conflicting results by saying that the positive responses were merely placebo effects – the products of wishful thinking by parents or physicians whose objectivity has been overcome by the desire for good results.

I recognize the plausibility of that argument, but an equally plausible argument can be made that the negative results may be the consequence of the researchers' expectation that the secretin will not have beneficial effects, and

---

Reproduced by permission of Dr. Bernard Rimland 29

**Down Syndrome and Vitamin Therapy**

therefore their conclusions are driven by what may be called the "negative placebo effect." It is easy to shoot down a new treatment in a double-blind trial – just refuse to see change in either group.

Example: a Wall Street Journal article (March 10, 1999), cited a number of very positive reports from parents and physicians who had tried secretin on autistic children, and stated that a study by neurologist Michael Chez of Chicago had shown no benefit.

Shortly after the Wall Street Journal article appeared, I was approached by a mother whose child had been treated with secretin by Dr. Chez. She told me that her son had "just soared" after the treatment, and that his improvement was noted by everyone who came in contact with the child. A speech therapist who had recently tested the boy retested him and the difference was so great that the speech therapist, unaware of the secretin, was baffled and kept insisting that she must have made a mistake in the earlier assessment. When the mother brought the child back to Dr. Chez's office, the office staff remarked that the boy had better eye contact and had obviously improved. Nevertheless, this mother was told by Dr. Chez that he could see no improvement, and it was just her wishful thinking that led her to believe the child had improved. Victoria Beck also was contacted by several mothers with similar stories.

Recently Chez and his co-workers published their study in the Journal of Autism and Developmental Disorders. They reported that the results were negative, that that they had seen no benefit from secretin.

In my commentary on the article, I pointed out that even though the research had many deficiencies, including the use of a very insensitive means of measuring improvement in the autistic children, the findings, contrary to the authors' declaration, were really quite positive. A number of significant differences were found, all favoring those given the secretin.

In a study recently published in the *New England Journal of Medicine*, Adrian Sandler et al. reported that they found no benefit from the administration of secretin to a sample of autistic children. Yet these authors also reported that 69% of the parents wanted their children to be continued on the secretin, even after they had been told that the study supposedly showed no benefit from the secretin. I have spoken to several mothers whose children were in that study, and was told that they have continued the secretin in their autistic children, with outstanding results.

In another study, Jennifer R. Lightdale et al. evaluated 20 autistic children for language skills and behaviour before and after receiving secretin. No control group was used. The researchers reported no differences in the children's ability either to understand speech or to express themselves. However, 15 of 18 parents said they saw moderate to significant improvement in the language skills of their autistic children following the secretin infusion.

Bruce Roseman and his colleagues conducted a secretin study on 10 children, to determine the effect on the children's behavior and language. A speech and language therapist, unaware of which children received secretin, tested the children. While the test results were supposedly negative, the speech therapist was able to correctly identify the children on the secretin 90% of the time.

In some of the studies cited above, the researchers acknowledged that their supposedly objective, scientific results conflicted with the observations of others, and agreed that further research is needed to help resolve these differences. Some also admitted that their single-dose studies were not conclusive; multi-dose studies have been started.

The negative placebo effect – bias in favor of seeing negative results – often hinges on the subjectivity of the measure employed, on the tendency to see the glass as half empty, versus half full; or to regard a 6-point difference on a rating scale as indicating trivial rather than worthwhile improvement.

In other cases, the negative placebo effect is built into the design or conduct of the study. For example, a recent study by Findling et al., evaluating vitamin B6 and magnesium as a treatment in Autism, neglected to include a "washout" period between the vitamin and placebo phases of the double-blind study. Apparently it was the authors' belief that since the B6 could not possibly have any beneficial effect, there was no need to include the usual several-week "washout" period in their study design. These authors also used unflavored vitamin B6, despite the fact that B6 is very bitter and most parents report that it is impossible to get their children to take unflavored B6. They did not use urine analysis to see if the vitamin had actually been consumed.

Similarly, in a study of vitamin B3 in Autism (vitamin B3 tastes even worse than vitamin B6), Greenbaum reported the children had taken unflavored vitamin B3 tablets. Many of the parents told me that their children had totally refused to take the tablets. The parents had complained to the study nurses, but the nurses just shrugged, and the study results were reported as though the children had taken the B3 and had shown no benefit. In fact, very few of them had consumed the vitamin.

The medical community looks with a jaundiced eye at reports that do not involve the use of placebo-controlled blind studies, dismissing them as merely anecdotal. I believe that the medical community should be looking with an equally jaundiced eye at controlled studies. The negative placebo effect – the expectation of and therefore the frequent finding of negative results by possibly biased researchers – is a problem that must be recognized if potentially useful treatments are to be properly evaluated and not prematurely rejected.

Dr. Bernard Rimland *Autism Research Review International*, 2000, Vol. 14, No. 2, pg 3

**Down Syndrome and Vitamin Therapy**

# Endnotes

1.  Howlin, P., Wing, L., and Gould, J. (1995) "The recognition of autism in children with Down syndrome: implications for intervention and some speculations about pathology." *Developmental Medicine and Child Neurology.* 37: 406-414.

2.  Kent, L., et al. (1999) "Comorbidity of autistic spectrum disorders in children with Down syndrome." *Developmental Medicine and Child Neurology* 41(3):,153-8

3.  Capone, G. (1999) "Down syndrome and Autistic spectrum disorder: a look at what we know." *Disability Solutions* 3(5&6): 8-15.

4.  Ghaziuddin, M., Tsai, L., and Gahziuddin, N. (1992) "Autism in Down's syndrome: presentation and diagnosis." *Journal of Intellectual Disability Research* 36: 449-456.

5.  Pary, R. (1997) "Comorbidity of Down syndrome and autism." *The Habilitative Mental Healthcare Newsletter.* 16(1).

6.  Pangborn, J., and Baker, S. (2001): *DEFEAT AUTISM NOW! Clinical Options Manual for Physicians.* Autism Research Institute, San Diego, CA.

7.  Knivsberg, A-M., et al. (1990) *Dietary Interventions in Autistic Syndromes. Brain Dysfunction* 3 (5-6): 315-327.

8.  Reichelt, K-L., et al. (1981) "Biologically Active Peptide Containing Fractions in Schizophrenia and Childhood Autism." *Advances in Biochemical Psychopharmacology* 28: 627-643

9.  Shattock, P., Lowdon, G. (1991) *Proteins, Peptides and Autism. Part 2: Implications for the Education and Care of People with Autism. Brain Dysfunction* 4(6): 323-334.

10. Reichelt, K-L., et al. (1990) "Gluten, milk proteins and autism: dietary intervention effects on behavior and peptide secretion." *Journal of Applied Nutrition* 42:1-8.

11. Knivsberg, A.M., Reichelt, K.L., Nødland, M. (2001) "Reports on dietary intervention in autistic disorders." *Nutritional Neuroscience.* 4(1):25-37.

12. Markus, C.R., et al. (2000) "The bovine protein alpha-lactalbumin increases the plasma ratio of tryptophan to the other large neutral amino acids, and in vulnerable subjects raises brain serotonin activity, reduces cortisol concentration, and improves mood under stress." *American Journal of Clinical Nutrition* 71: 1536-1544.

13. Markus, C.R., et al. (2002) "Whey protein rich in lactoferrin increases the ratio of plasma tryptophan to the sum of the other large neutral amino acids and improves cognitive performance in stress-vulnerable subjects." *American Journal of Clinical Nutrition* 75: 1051-1056.

14. http://www.autism.com/ari/contents.html

15. Kadrabova, J., et al. (1996) "Changed serum trace element profile in Down's syndrome." *Biological Trace Elements Research* 54: 201-206.

16. Walsh, W.J. (2002) *MT Protein and Its Role in Autism.* Presented at the 3rd International Medical Conference on Autism, Montreal, Canada.

17. Megson, M. "Is Autism a G-Alpha Protein Defect Reversible with Natural Vitamin A." *Medical Hypotheses* 54(6): 979-83.

18. Kane, P. (1999) "The Neurobiology of Lipids in Autistic Spectrum Disorder"*Journal of Orthomolecular Medicine* 14: 103.

19. James, S.J., et al. (1999) "Abnormal folate metabolism and mutation in the methylene-tetrahydrofolate reductase gene may be maternal risk factors for Down syndrome." *American Journal of Clinical Nutrition.* 70: 495-501.

20. Thien, K.R., et al. (1977) "Serum folates in man." *Journal of Clinical Pathology.* 30(5): 438-4.

21. Piven, J., and Palmer, P. (1999) "Psychiatric disorder and the broad autism phenotype: evidence from a family study of multiple-incidence autism families." *American Journal of Psychiatry,* 156 (4): 557-563.

22. Baumgartner, E.R., et al. (1985) "Comparison of folic acid coenzyme distribution patterns in patients with methylenetetrahydrofolate reductase and methionine synthase deficiencies." *Pediatric Research* 19(12):.1288-92

23. Bernard, S.R. "Metabolic Models for Methyl and Inorganic Mercury." *Health Phys.* 46(12) 1415-1419. Dec. 1986.

24. http://commons.ucalgary.ca/mercury/

25. Horvath, K., et al. (1998) "Improved social and language skills after secretin administration in patients with autistic spectrum disorders." *Journal of the Association for Academic Minority Physicians* 9(1): 9-15.

26. Horvath, K., et al. (1999) "Gastrointestinal abnormalities in children with autistic disorder." *Journal of Pediatrics* 135(5): 559-63.

27. Owley, T., et al. (1999) "A double-blind, placebo-controlled trial of secretin for the treatment of autistic disorder." http://www.medscape.com/Medscape/GeneralMedicine/journal/1999/v01.n10/mgm1006.owle/mgm1006.owle01.html

28. Sandler, A., et al. (1999) "Lack of benefit of a single dose of synthetic human secretin in the treatment of autism and pervasive developmental disorder." *New England Journal of Medicine* 341: 1801-6.

29. Rimland, Dr. Bernard (1999) "Secretin update: a negative placebo effect?" *Autism Research Review International* Vol. 14, No. 2, p. 3

30. Rimland, Dr. Bernard (1999) "Secretin: positive, negative reports in the 'top of the inning'." *Autism Research Review International* Vol. 13, No. 4, p. 7

**Down Syndrome and Vitamin Therapy**

# CLARA'S STORY

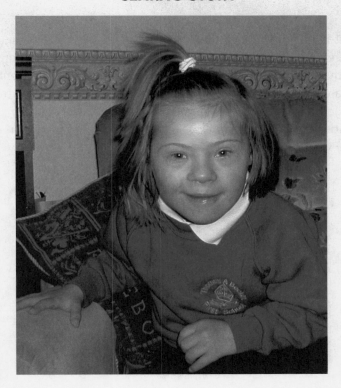

As the youngest of four children, Clara White leads an active life. A busy four-year-old, Clara attends pre-school near her home in Worthing, a seaside town on the south coast of England. Her mother, Hazel, says that games are one of Clara's favourite pastimes.

"Clara loves playing picture lotto and memory games. She seems to have a good memory which I'm sure is due to the vitamins she takes as children like Clara often have bad memory. She sleeps well at night and has been out of nappies since she was two, which I also think has been helped by the vitamins she takes. Clara was a very chesty baby and suffered with a lot of colds and high temperatures. Since she started taking the MSB vitamins, her colds have become less frequent. In the last twelve months, she had only one."

Hazel is so convinced in the power of Nutri-Chem's MSB formula for children with Down Syndrome that she now works as local supplier to other parents in England and Europe. "I think it's important if you are going to take this type of formula, or any vitamins, that you get it from a source like Nutri-Chem. They have studied nutritional supplements for children with Down Syndrome for many years."

# CHAPTER 5

# UNDERSTANDING ANTIBIOTICS AND EAR INFECTIONS

*I OFTEN SPEAK AT CONFERENCES for parents of children with Down Syndrome. At one such conference recently, a medical doctor told parents that nutritional supplements are useless for their children. A mother in the audience said her child was constantly sick and on antibiotics repeatedly, yet her child didn't improve. What, she asked, could she do? The medical response she received: "See your doctor."*

*I could see this mother's frustration at such an answer, since it was her doctor who was prescribing the antibiotics in the first place.*

*The fact is, antibiotics are over-prescribed in North America and when they're used inappropriately, antibiotics are making people sicker. Parents need more information about antibiotics: their uses, abuses and alternatives.*
*– K.M.*

## WHAT WILL I LEARN?

▸ Why antibiotics may cause more problems than they solve.

▸ Why doctors prescribe unnecessary antibiotics.

▸ How you can support your child's health without antibiotics.

▸ The link between ear infections and learning.

In nature, there's a universal law that all living things are related. As humans, we're beginning to understand these relationships as they exist in our environment and within our own bodies. It's pretty basic: if you interfere with the natural order of things, and remove one thing, something else will take its place to fill the void you've created. If a farmer kills all the foxes that are threatening the chickens, he'll end up with too many rabbits. It seems that in traditional medicine this law of nature has been forgotten when it comes to antibiotics.

**DEFINING MOMENT**

**Bacteria:** Single-celled organisms that are found in food, air, soil and the human body. Good bacteria prevent infections. Other bacteria cause disease.

**Virus:** Infectious, disease-causing particles that reproduce by invading and taking over living cells; virus is Latin for poison.

**Fungi:** Multi-cellular microorganisms that are universally distributed and include molds, mushrooms, mildews. Some are harmful to plants and animals, including humans, while some fungi are valued as food or for the fermentations that they produce (for example yeast and beer).

## The good, the bad, and the inappropriate

Antibiotics are chemical drugs used to kill bacterial infections such as strep throat and some sinus, bladder and lung infections. Antibiotics are not effective for viral infections. These include bronchitis, colds, influenza and ear infections.[1]

Widespread publication of the harmful effects of antibiotics has made people rightfully suspicious of their use. We're seeing growing rates of antibiotic-resistant infections such as influenzas.

Consider what happened with tuberculosis. In the 1940s, scientists discovered the first of several drugs now used to treat TB. TB began to disappear, and in the 1960s it was brought under tight control. However, federal funding for TB-prevention and control efforts was reduced, and this has had disastrous effects. By 1984, the incidence of TB began to rise again in the U.S. TB remains the leading infectious cause of death worldwide, claiming two to three million lives annually, mainly in countries with limited health facilities.

Due to interruptions in drug supply, improper drug prescriptions and nonadherence to treatment protocols, multi-drug resistant (MDR) TB strains are now prevalent in society. Although TB was once very successfully treated with medication (i.e. to the point where TB was almost eliminated in the U.S.), the success rate with MDR strains is limited. A study done in China found that only 80% of MDR TB cases were treatable.[2]

Drug-resistant strains of bacteria often develop when antibiotics are incorrectly prescribed or are not taken long enough. (This last situation happens frequently with antibiotics. There's an initial decrease in symptoms and, thinking you're no longer sick, you stop taking the drug.) When you take an antibiotic, it kills bacteria – both the infection-causing strains as well as the disease-fighting ones. So you have fewer defenses against future infection. If not all of the infection-causing bacteria is destroyed, the survivors can mutate into ones that can resist the antibiotic. A rebound infection occurs, one that has already proven itself immune to the antibiotic. If more and stronger antibiotics are used, it increases the vicious cycle of disease.

Ear infections are one of the most common reasons for antibiotic use in children. Studies now show that antibiotic use for ear infections is often unnecessary since most infections clear up regardless of the type of treatment.[3] Researchers report that nearly two-thirds of children with uncomplicated ear infections recover from pain and fever within 24 hours and more than 80% recover within seven days.[4] In fact, some governments are funding educational programs to ensure that children do not receive antibiotics as a matter of course. In some cases, school officials are sending information home with students that educates parents about the appropriate use of antibiotics and the dangers of overuse.

## If it's so bad, why do they do it?

Almost half (44%) of children seen by their doctor for a common cold leave with a prescription for unnecessary antibiotics, reported the *Journal of the American Medical Association* in March 1998.5 Knowing the harmful side-effects antibiotics can cause, researchers are now looking at the reasons for their over-prescription. What they're finding is that:

### The immune connection

Children with Down Syndrome have more food allergies which can exhibit symptoms that look like ear infections. One of the most common foods in any child's diet is milk. Removing milk and dairy products completely for one month will give an indication of whether or not milk products are an issue. Other food and food groups can also cause problems and lab testing or removal of certain foods can help determine sources of trouble.

- physicians may not know that antibiotics are useless in viral infections (71% of family physicians reported that they would immediately prescribe an antibiotic to a child with one day of light nasal discharge and a low-grade fever);

- physicians use antibiotics for prevention despite no evidence that supports such use;

- patients expect to receive a prescription for antibiotics based on past experience;

- economic pressures on physicians demand that they see more patients and spend less time with them on such things as patient education.

# Stop the train, I want to get off

If you're concerned about antibiotic overuse, take these steps:

- Parents must insist on better diagnosis from their physicians before accepting a prescription for antibiotics. If an ear infection is caused by inflammation or allergies, deal with the cause and not the symptom. In some cases, ear tubes may be a preferable solution because of the harm antibiotics can do. Dietary changes may be necessary.

- Natural immune-boosters may prove effective against infection. These include vitamins A, C and E, and the minerals zinc and selenium. The herb echinacea has also proven to be beneficial.[6, 7, 8, 9, 10, 11, 12, 13]

- You can also use probiotics as a preventative measure. Probiotics are essentially live bacteria that survive passage through the gastrointestinal tract and have beneficial effects on the host.[14]

- Don't accept prophylactic antibiotics (preventative antibiotics). They don't work and can create rebound infections.

> ## The candida connection
>
> Antibiotic use often results in candida, a yeast infection where the healthy bacteria (lactobacillus, acidophilus) that normally keep the Candida Albicans yeast in a healthy balance are killed off by the antibiotic. This yeast, which lives in the vagina, mouth and intestines, then reproduces to the point of infection. Short-term treatment involves use of acidophilus supplements. A healthy immune system is the best long-term defense.

# Ear infections and learning ability

When a child is sick, his or her ability to learn is reduced. Frequent ear infections in infancy are associated with developmental delay and lower I.Q. scores.[16] It has been reported that children with Down Syndrome who do not have ear infections do better in language ability than those suffering with ear infections.[17] In fact, only 18% of children with Down Syndrome who had untreated ear infections achieved the median language ability when compared to other children with Down Syndrome. Of the control group who had not had infections, 65% achieved median language developments.[18] This clearly demonstrates how illness can affect learning. (It should also be noted that there are significant financial costs associated with ear infections: one study found that the cost to parents for lost work time associated with ear infection-related child care was $1,157 U.S..[19])

## Probiotics – nature's good guys

When the healthy bacteria in your body have been destroyed by disease or antibiotics, probiotics can restore the balance. They are live bacteria that survive passage through the gastrointestinal tract and have beneficial effects on the host.

Unlike antibiotics which kill bacteria, probiotics work by restoring the good bacteria your body needs. Probiotics can be used in place of antibiotics in some cases, or to restore the good bacteria which antibiotics have destroyed. Studies are showing positive benefits from probiotics in lowering blood pressure and cholesterol, treating allergies and controlling lactose intolerance.

It is possible to obtain probiotics from yogurt and fermented foods, but it's difficult unless the specific strain of necessary bacteria is present (which is not the case in most commercial yogurt).[15]

# Closing comments from Kent:

A major newspaper recently did an investigative article about how much money drug companies lavish on physicians in an attempt to persuade them of the benefits of their drug products. This enraged readers. What enrages me is something else instead. When I speak to doctors, they tell me that they're very independent-minded when it comes to choosing which antibiotic to prescribe to patients.

These doctors are missing the point. They've forfeited the game before the starting whistle even blows. What I find outrageous isn't whether or not they make up their own minds about which antibiotic to use – it's that they show no awareness of proven antibiotic alternatives. – K.M.

## If antibiotics are required...

Acidophilus will reduce the side effects of antibiotics. If an antibiotic is necessary, using acidophilus along with it will restore the "good" bacteria that helps digestion and suppress undesirable bacteria and yeast (candida). Acidophilus should be taken between doses of the antibiotic, not at the same time, because the antibiotic can kill off the acidophilus bacteria. Be sure to refrigerate your acidophilus to keep this good bacteria alive.

I recommend Nutridophilus brand of acidophilus because the storage and delivery is strictly controlled, thereby ensuring potency. Virtually all strains of bacteria lose most of their benefit if left unrefrigerated for several months. Nutridophilus is also enteric coated. Because acidophilus is sensitive to acid in the stomach, enteric coating protects the acidophilus from this stomach acid and releases it in the bowel, a safer environment for bacteria.

# Endnotes

1.  Nyquist, A-C., et al. (1998) "Antibiotic prescribing for children with colds, upper respiratory tract infections, and bronchitis." *Journal of the American Medical Association* 279: 875-877.

2.  Long, R. (2000) "Drug-resistant tuberculosis. *Canadian Medical Association Journal* 163(4): 425-8.; Yew, W.W., et al. (2000) "Outcomes of patients with multidrug-resistant pulmonary tuberculosis treated with ofloxacin/ levofloxacin-containing regimens." *Chest* 117(3): 744-51.; Centers for Disease Control, Atlanta www.cdc.gov

3.  Damoiseaux, R., et al. (2000) "Primary care based randomised, double blind trial of amoxicillin versus placebo for acute otitis media in children aged under 2 years" *British Medical Journal* 320:350-4; Williams, R.L., et al. (1993) "Use of antibiotics in preventing recurrent acute otitis media and in treating otitis media with effusion. A meta-analytic attempt to resolve the brouhaha." *Journal of the American Medical Association* 270(11):1344-51.

4.  Agency for Healthcare Research and Quality, Rockville, MD, August 9, 2000

5.  Nyquist, A-C., et al. (1998) "Antibiotic prescribing for children with colds, upper respiratory tract infections, and bronchitis." *Journal of the American Medical Association* 279: 875-77.

6.  Bjorksten, B., et al. (1980) "Zinc and immune function in Down's syndrome." *Acta Paediatrica Scand* 69: 183-187.

7.  Fabris, N., et al. (1993) "Psychoendocrine – immune interactions in Down's syndrome: Role of zinc." In: *Growth Hormone Treatment in Down's syndrome* (ed. S. Castells and K.E. Wisniewski, John Wiley & Sons Ltd, London) p203-217.

8.  Franceschi, C., et al. (1988) "Oral zinc supplementation in Down's syndrome: restoration of thymic endocrine activity and of some immune defects." *Journal of Mental Deficiency Research* 32: 169-181.

9.  Lockitch, G., et al. (1989) "Infection and immunity in Down syndrome: A trial of long-term low oral doses of zinc." *Journal of Pediatrics* 114: 781-7.

10. Anneren, G., et al. (1990) "Increase in serum concentrations of IgG2 and IgG4 by selenium supplementation in children with Down's syndrome." *Archives of Disease in Childhood* 65: 1353-1355.

11. Meydani, S., et al. (1997) "Vitamin E supplementation and in vivo immune response in healthy elderly subjects." *Journal of the American Medical Association* 277: 1380-86.

12. Chandra, R. (1992) "Effect of vitamin and trace-element supplementation on immune responses and infection in elderly subjects." *Lancet* 340: 1124-27.

13. Pike, J., and Chandra, R.K. (1995) "Effect of vitamin and trace element supplementation on immune indices in healthy elderly." *International Journal of Vitamin and Nutritional Research* 65: 117-20.

14. Gates, G. (1999) "Otitis media – the pharyngeal connection." *Journal of the American Medical Association.* 282: 987-89.

15. Collins, M.D., and Gibson, G.R. (1999) "Probiotics, prebiotics, and synbiotics: approaches for modulating the microbial ecology of the gut." *American Journal of Clinical Nutrition* 69(suppl): 1052S-7S; de Roos, N.M. and Katan, M.B. (2000) "Effects of probiotic bacteria on diarrhea, lipid metabolism, and carcinogenesis: a review of papers published between 1988 and 1998." *American Journal of Clinical Nutrition* 71(2): 405-411.

16. Gates, G. (1999) "Otitis media – the pharyngeal connection." *Journal of the American Medical Association.* 282: 987-89.

17. Whiteman, B., et al. (1986) "Relationship of otitis media and language impairment in adolescents with Down syndrome." *Mental Retardation* 24: 353-6.

18. Rolfe, R. (2000) "The role of probiotic culture in the control of gastrointestinal health." *Journal of Nutrition* 130: 396S-402S.

19. Alsarraf, R. (98) *Meeting of the American Society of Pediatric Otolaryngology.*

# MICHAEL'S STORY

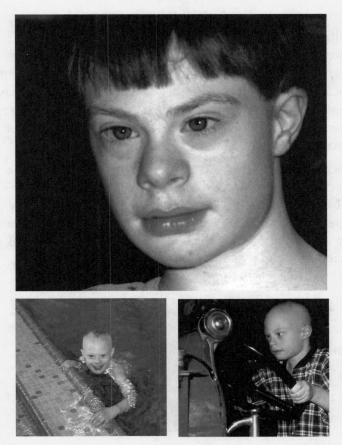

If there's one thing 13-year-old Michael Leger can't stand, it's doctor's visits and tests. So when his mother, Patty, decided it was time to do something about his alopecia – an immune disorder causing hair loss – she thought it was time to give alternative treatment a try. She knew about vitamin therapies for children with Down Syndrome, but had been put off by the polarization among parents over the issue. "There were two groups. You were either for it or against it."

Despite the controversy, Patty was concerned about her son's increasing baldness. His hair loss had been patchy for six years, but by the age of nine Michael was completely bald. Conventional medical treatments involved tests and drugs such as cortisone. Because of Michael's aversion to doctor's visits and Patty's own reservations about using drugs for the problem, she ruled out this approach.

"I became interested in vitamin therapy after reading that alopecia was a problem of oxidation and the immune system, and I found out that this was part of Nutri-Chem's MSB formula. Our pediatrician said that vitamin therapy might not work, but to go ahead and try it. Within six months of starting on MSB, Michael's hair had regrown. After six years of losing his hair, it was too coincidental that it stopped with the vitamins."

# CHAPTER 6

# DRUGS AND DOWN SYNDROME

IN PHARMACOLOGY, THERE IS A CONCEPT called the "therapeutic window." It indicates how well a drug works versus how safe it is. Where vitamins are concerned, the therapeutic window is wide: a broad range of benefits without risk.

When it comes to drugs, some have a narrow therapeutic window: specific benefit, great risk. There is a saying that because so many drugs have been approved for safety only to be withdrawn later because of harmful effects, you have to "hurry up and take it while it's proven safe."

Many variables affect the way our bodies handle drugs: age, metabolic proficiency, airways and how well our kidneys, liver and bowel function. In children who have Down Syndrome, there is a high incidence of thyroid problems which affect metabolism. Bowel function, also a problem in many children with Down Syndrome, is an essential elimination tool for drugs.

**WHAT WILL I LEARN?**

▸ How to consider risk and benefit in treatment choices.

▸ The special drug risks faced by people with Down Syndrome.

▸ The benefits and risks of vitamins versus drugs.

At Nutri-Chem, I routinely hear of children with Down Syndrome being prescribed drugs for which the safety and effect are largely unproven, for instance, psychoactive drugs such as Ritalin and Prozac. There is no doubt that some drugs save lives and others may be of benefit with little or no risk.

*It is my role as a pharmacist to educate parents and health professionals on the effectiveness of the drug, the risk of taking the drug and the third dimension which is the corporate bias which tends to support patented drug therapy over natural non-patentable therapy.*

*Some of our MSB customers have chosen to use drugs they believe will improve their child's intelligence or growth. Our job at Nutri-Chem is to support these families, and all our MSB users, by providing nutritional information and effective, safe supplements that minimize health problems and help children achieve optimal health. – K.M.*

## The cure can be worse than the disease

Of 250,00 hospital deaths in one year in the U.S., 106,000 were attributed to "non-error, negative effects of drugs," Dr. Barbara Starfield of the Johns Hopkins School of Hygiene and Public Health reported in an article published in July, 2000 in the Journal of the American Medical Association.[1] This statistic is alarming because these were drugs that were prescribed properly, for the proper condition, that led to these 106,000 deaths in hospitals alone! What was not considered were properly prescribed drug-related deaths that occurred outside of hospitals in the community. This *JAMA* study concludes that errors caused by the medical system is the third leading cause of death in the United States. Pharmacists, patients and their doctors should all work together to reduce such appalling statistics. Awareness of this situation is the first step.

Then there is the issue of drug regulation: is it adequate to ensure safety and effectiveness in the face of corporate-sponsored testing and promotion with vast profits at stake?

# Special concerns for Down Syndrome

Children with Down Syndrome have a higher incidence of many conditions and diseases (ear infections, bowel problems, hypothyroidism, Autism and leukemia) for which drugs are prescribed. In addition, some parents have sought to increase intelligence or change stature with the use of drugs. Because of the often-considerable side effects and potential harm that drugs may present, combined with alterations in some important cycles in the body from the presence of an extra chromosome, it is essential that parents become educated about the benefits and risks of drugs.

Issues for children with Down Syndrome can be related to physical differences inherent in the genetic disorder. For example, there is greater likelihood of obstructed airways for these children. There are also obvious metabolic differences which suggest more sensitivity to certain drugs

## Biotransformation and elimination of drugs

Many drugs are lipid-soluble (lipophilic), weak organic acids or bases that are not readily eliminated from the body. To be excreted more rapidly, they must be transformed into more water-soluble (hydrophilic) compounds.

Biotransformation is classified into two phases:
Phase 1: Oxidation, Reduction and Hydrolysis
Phase 2: Conjugation with activated sulfate, activated glucoronic acid, activated acetic acid, amino acids.

In phase 1 reaction the molecule of the drug is changed, and in phase 2 reactions something is added to the molecule, in both cases to render a more water-soluble molecule.

The enzyme system of the liver is responsible for the biotransformation of the majority of drugs and nutrients. Other tissues are kidney, lung, plasma and the gastrointestinal tract.

Drugs absorbed from the intestines are transported to the liver right away and are thus subject to the so-called "first-pass effect" which represents the combined action of gastrointestinal, epithelial and hepatic drug metabolizing enzyme.

In addition, if the amino acids necessary for the above mentioned phase 2 reactions, like glycine, glutamine and glutathione, are missing, the body's detox-function is compromised.

(including atropine and methotrexate). Because of depleted glutathione in children with Down Syndrome, there can be difficulty in certain drugs being cleared from the body.

## Drugs of concern in Down Syndrome

**ANESTHESIA AND OTHER SEDATIVES:** In Down Syndrome, there is a higher incidence of narrow airways, altered respiratory function and gastro-reflux. When you give anesthetic or sedative drugs to children with Down Syndrome, there is a higher risk of adverse effects. Impaired drug clearance found in children with Down Syndrome can result in the effects of sedatives and anesthetics being magnified.[2, 3, 4, 5] Parents should speak with the anesthetist or doctor in charge so they are aware of these potential risks. Also, if your child is having any type of surgery, inform the doctor and pharmacist of any vitamin, herbal and other medications your child is taking.

**ARICEPT:** An anti-cholinergic drug that prevents the breakdown of acetylcholine, a neurotransmitter needed for brain cells to communicate with one another. This drug, developed for people with Alzheimer's disease, has shown to have short-term benefits, but many side effects.[6, 7]

**ATROPINE:** Used pre-operatively to dry up membranes during surgery. Children with Down Syndrome have an increased sensitivity to atropine possibly due to depleted storage of the neurotransmitter acetylcholine in the brain. This increases side effects such as tremors, flushing, dryness, mood alterations and agitation.[8]

**GROWTH HORMONE:** Medically, growth hormones are used for thyroid problems. The hypothalamus and pituitary glands make Thyroid Stimulating Hormones (TSH) which control thyroid function, and are involved in normal growth and development. Controversy arises when growth hormone is used for growth enhancement alone in children with normal thyroid function.[9, 10, 11, 12]

**METHOTREXATE:** This drug is an anti-folate which is used in the treatment of cancer to inhibit DNA production needed for cell production and growth. Because folate metabolism in children with Down Syndrome is already altered (known as functional folate deficiency, discussed in *Chapter 12: One Mother's Story*), children treated with methotrexate experience greater sensitivity to negative effects of the drug and may suffer neurological damage.[13, 14, 15, 16, 17, 18] (Please refer to *Chapter 12* for complete details.)

**PIRACETAM:** A nootropic drug (a class of drugs that act as cognitive enhancers) that is believed to improve learning and memory. Small studies have shown benefits of piracetam in Down Syndrome and Dyslexia. Other small studies have shown no benefits to piracetam in Down Syndrome. Anecdotally, parents have reported significant benefits for their children with Down Syndrome. At this point it would be difficult to say whether there is enough evidence favouring or against the use of piracetam in Down Syndrome.[19, 20] (Please refer to *Appendix A: Existing Studies and their Limitations* for more details on piracetam.)

---

# Closing comments from Kent:

*One of the main criticisms against the use of vitamins for children with Down Syndrome is that their benefits haven't been tested on these children. For example, vitamin E is now accepted for use in destroying free radicals which damage the brain. Children with Down Syndrome exhibit free radical brain damage before the age of 40. Yet despite the safety of vitamin E supplements, it is not recommended based on the lack of studies on vitamin E with kids with Down Syndrome. Contrast this with the widespread and often casual use of a great variety of drugs whose use on people with Down Syndrome has also not been studied. In my view, given the great risk drugs represent and their uselessness in the face of many conditions, this practice is questionable at best. – K.M.*

# Endnotes

1.  Starfield, B. (2000) "Is US Health Really the Best in the World?" *Journal of the American Medical Association* 284(4): 483-85.

2.  Butler, M.G., et al. (2000) "Specific genetic diseases at risk for sedation/anesthesia complications." *Anesthesia and Analgesia*. 91(4):,83.

3.  Shott, S.R. (2000) "Down syndrome: analysis of airway size and a guide for appropriate intubation." *Laryngoscope*. 110(4):.585-92.

4.  Kobel, M., et al. (1982) "Anaesthetic considerations in Down's syndrome: experience with 100 patients and a review of the literature." *Canadian Anaesthetists' Society Journal*. 29(6): 593-9.

5.  Napoli, K.L., et al. (1996) "Safety and efficacy of chloral hydrate sedation in children undergoing echocardiography." *Journal of Pediatrics*. 129(2): 287-91.

6.  Kishnani, P.S., et al.(1999) "Cholinergic therapy for Down's syndrome." *Lancet* 353(9158): 1064-5.

7.  Hemingway-Eltomey, J.M., Lerner, A.J. (1999) "Adverse effects of donepezil in treating Alzheimer's disease associated with Down's syndrome" (letter). *American Journal of Psychiatry* 156: 1470.

8.  http://drugs.medbroadcast.com/ASP/DrugInfo.asp?BrandNameID=871

9.  Anneren, G., et al. (2000) "Growth hormone therapy in young children with Down syndrome and a clinical comparison of Down and Prader-Willi syndromes." *Growth Hormone and IGF Research*. 10 Suppl B:S87-91.

10. Anneren, G., et al. (1999) "Growth hormone treatment in young children with Down's syndrome: effects on growth and psychomotor development." *Archives of Disease in Childhood*. 80(4): 334-8.

11. Castells, S., et al. (1996) "Hypothalamic versus pituitary dysfunction in Down's syndrome as cause of growth retardation." *Journal of Intellectual Disability Research*. 40(Pt 6): 509-17.

12. Kodish, E., Cuttler, L., (1996) "Ethical issues in emerging new treatments such as growth hormone therapy for children with Down syndrome and Prader-Willi syndrome." *Current Opinion in Pediatrics*. 8(4): 401-5.

13. Rubin, C.M., Mick, R., Johnson, F.L. (1996) "Bone marrow transplantation for the treatment of haematological disorders in Down's syndrome: toxicity and outcome." *Bone Marrow Transplantation*. 18(3):533-40.

14. Peeters, M.A., et al. (1995) "In vivo folic acid supplementation partially corrects in vitro methotrexate toxicity in patients with Down syndrome." *British Journal of Haematology* 89(3): 678-80.

15. Kalwinsky, D.K., et al. (1990) "Clinical and biological characteristics of acute lymphocytic leukemia in children with Down syndrome." *American Journal of Medical Genetics Supplement*. 7:267-71

16. Lejeune, J. (1990) "Pathogenesis of mental deficiency in trisomy 21." *American Journal of Medical Genetics Supplement.* 7:20-30.

17. Garre, M.L., et al. (1987) "Pharmacokinetics and toxicity of methotrexate in children with Down syndrome and acute lymphocytic leukemia." *Journal of Pediatrics* 111(4): 606-12.

18. Peeters, M., Poon, A. (1987) "Down syndrome and leukemia: unusual clinical aspects and unexpected methotrexate sensitivity." *European Journal of Pediatrics.* 146(4): 416-22.

19. Vampirelli, P. (1978) [Piracetam in child neuropsychiatry. Clinical experimentation in a child neuropsychiatry department]. *Minerva Pediatrica.* 30(4): 373-6. Italian.

20. Lobaugh, N.J., et al. (2001) "Piracetam therapy does not enhance cognitive functioning in children with down syndrome." *Archives of Pediatric and Adolescent Medicine.* 155(4): 442-8.

# SECTION 2
# THE TRADITIONAL APPROACH

### CHAPTER 5
#### UNDERSTANDING ANTIBIOTICS AND EAR INFECTIONS

### CHAPTER 6
#### DRUGS AND DOWN SYNDROME

# MOLLY AND MEGAN'S STORY

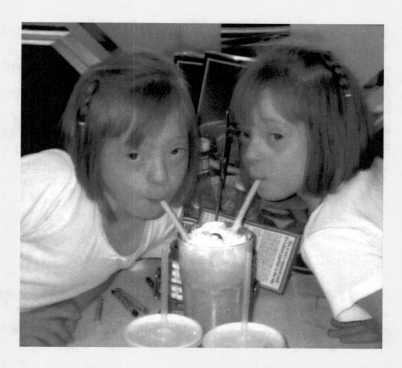

Kim Myers didn't find out her twin daughters had Down Syndrome until they were six months old. "Their pediatrician said he had suspected it when they were three months, but simply put the information in his files with a note that he 'didn't want to disrupt our family's lives'," Kim recalls. "I had no earthly idea about Down Syndrome. I had never known anyone who had it."

However, once she heard the news, Kim did some research on the Internet and found out about vitamin therapy and MSB. "There was no question that's what we wanted for Molly and Megan even though the doctor said no way. I'm aggressive, outspoken, don't take no for an answer, and I want answers quickly." As a result, Kim did two things: she ordered MSB from Nutri-Chem, and she fired the pediatrician.

Now turning five, Molly and Megan have a doctor who accepts that "they will always be on vitamins and piracetam," says Kim. And while he doesn't always agree with her, she says "he does think that the girls are doing awesome."

With no health problems, Molly and Megan are turning five as pin-up girls: they've been featured several times in their city's children's calendar. Kim says they have lots of energy and love creative play. "I've read so many books that say children with Down Syndrome can't do imaginative play, but Molly and Megan always have," Kim says. The girls and younger brother Jake (who also takes vitamins) have a healthy diet – lots of fruit and vegetables, no soda pop and very little sugar.

"I can't tell you how many times people come up to me and say Molly and Megan are so active, and just like children who don't have Down Syndrome. I'm asked all the time what we're doing that makes them so healthy and bright. My reason for giving them nutritional supplements is preventative. I can't believe people who don't want to do something that makes a child's life so much better. Molly and Megan are graduating from their pre-school, and everybody there is so sad to see them leave for public school. They are going to be so awesome there, and they will be teaching others."

# CHAPTER 7

# THE DIGESTIVE SYSTEM

*I HAVE WORKED WITH MANY CHILDREN with Down Syndrome and Autism and their parents. In my work, I found that when I was able to improve bowel function in a child with Autism, mental function improved. The bowel is so important because it affects the brain and the immune system. It digests and absorbs nutrients and is a primary organ for toxin and waste removal. Because of my many years of "dedication" to the bowel, the parents at the Giant Steps School for Autism presented me with a children's book on the bowel inscribed to Kent MacLeod, Dr. Poop! – K.M.*

**WHAT WILL I LEARN?**

▶ The five keys to healthy digestion.

▶ The connection between bowel health and the overall health of your immune system.

▶ How one extra chromosome affects digestive processes for people with Down Syndrome.

# The healthy digestive system
## Keep your body in running order

A nutrient-rich diet, properly digested and absorbed for use in the body, is the best defense against illness and disease. If you think of your body as a car, the best way to avoid costly repairs and breakdowns is to keep the car in good running order: use high octane gas, change your oil and filter regularly and keep the spark plugs, brakes and battery from wearing out so the car doesn't end up on the scrap heap before its time. In your body, good quality food, properly functioning organs, enzymes and healthy bacteria and a healthy waste removal system ensure health and longevity.

## Digestion: a trip with stops along the way

When we say digestion, most of us probably think that it's something that happens in our stomachs. In fact, digestion is a process that starts as you bite into your food, and doesn't end until waste is eliminated from the body.

Digestion begins in your mouth. You bite into a sandwich and start chewing, causing the initial breakdown of food. Saliva gets into the act, adding moisture to the mix. You swallow the now-mushy sandwich and it passes down the esophagus to your

### DEFINING MOMENT

### Amino acids:

Known as the "building blocks" of life, amino acids are critically important. Protein in the food we eat is broken down into amino acids. The body then builds the proteins it needs as part of every cell in our bodies. Some amino acids are also involved as neurotransmitters which carry nerve impulses from one cell to another. In other words, they're needed to send and receive messages from the brain. Other amino acids work helping vitamins and minerals to function.

Some amino acids are called **non-essential.** What this really means (because they ARE essential) is that they can be made in our body. The remaining (called **essential**) have to come from our food or from supplements. Following are definitions of the role played by individual essential and non-essential amino acids.

stomach. Here digestive enzymes and gastric juices go to work, and begin the breakdown of fats. Then, it passes to the next stop on the journey: the duodenum (the first section of the small intestine).

Digestive enzymes from your pancreas and bile from your liver (stored in the gall bladder) act on the now-liquid material, called chyme, in the duodenum. These enzymes continue the breakdown of fats, starches and proteins, and as a result of the protein digestion, amino acids are released. As the food enters your small intestine, enzymes from pancreatic and intestinal juices continue the digestion of fats and proteins. Special intestinal enzymes break down starches and carbohydrates into simple sugars (glucose, galactose and fructose).

Your small intestine has a major function in the digestive process, and is also the most important organ of absorption, as digested food is distributed through the blood and lymphatic system for use by your body. The rate at which your food is converted to energy (while breathing, sleeping, sitting) is controlled by thyroid hormone, which is produced by your thyroid gland.

## Essential Amino Acids

(must be supplied in the diet or from supplements):

**ARGININE** is essential during the growth period, but can subsequently be manufactured in the body. It is synthesized in a series of reactions involving ornithine, cirtulline, aspartic and glutamic acids in the urea cycle. Arginine has a vital role in the urea cycle.

**HISTIDINE** is used in the maintenance of myelin sheaths. Histidine is a precursor to histamine, which acts as a stimulus for stomach acid secretion and is released in allergic reactions. It is also essential for zinc and copper regulation.

**LEUCINE** is mainly utilized by muscle for the formation of alanine.

**LYSINE** is important for the formation of collagen in a process regulated by vitamin C. Without vitamin C or adequate lysine, wounds will not heal properly and susceptibility to infection will increase. Lysine also functions to ensure adequate absorption of calcium. Carnitine (involved in transporting fatty acids across the mitochondria) is derived from lysine.

Material that was not digested and absorbed ends up in your large intestine (colon). Here the water is absorbed and the solid material (feces) leaves your body through the anus.

### Essential Amino Acids cont.

**METHIONINE** belongs to the family of sulfur-containing amino acids (cysteine, taurine). Sulfer amino acids serve as natural carriers of the trace element selenium and have roles in protection (ie antioxidants) and detoxification. Methionine functions as a methyl donor and a precursor to the other sulfur-containing amino acids. Methionine is needed for the formation of carnitine and creatinine and helps maintain the liver's production of lecithin.

**PHENYLALANINE** is a precursor of many neurotransmitters including dopamine, norepinephrine and epinephrine and to thyroid hormones. Tyrosine is derived from phenylalanine.

**THREONINE** can be catabolized to pyruvate or acetyle CoA and is important for energy metabolism. The primary pathway for threonine catabolism requires vitamin B6.

# When it works
## Synergy is everything

The basic rule of nutritional science is that of synergy. Everything is inter-related, with nutrients co-dependent on others, not working in isolation. Our bodies function in much the same way. In a healthy body, all of the parts work together. For food to be digested and absorbed and waste eliminated, all organs and processes must be working. Healthy intestinal bacteria and digestive enzymes act as a waste treatment plant, filtering out toxins and producing clean material for our body's use.

# When it breaks down
## Problems we all face

This book is about Down Syndrome, yet the very illnesses and diseases prevalent in this genetic disorder are increasing at alarming rates in North America. This is especially true of conditions related to the bowel. Irritable bowel syndrome, unheard of just a few years ago, is rampant. Celiac disease, Crohn's disease, lactose and gluten intolerance, food allergies, gastrointestinal infections and constipation/diarrhea: all are now becoming commonplace conditions in people of all ages.

Some examples:

- Recent research points to a bowel link in Attention Deficit Disorder, hypothyroidism and Autism, conditions which are also showing huge increases in the general population. For people with Autism, inflammation of several areas of the GI tract are frequently reported, and chronic diarrhea, gaseousness and abdominal discomfort are common.[1] The bowel and Autism are discussed thoroughly in *Chapter 4: Autism and Down Syndrome.*

> **Essential Amino Acids cont.**
>
> **TRYPTOPHAN** affects neuro-transmitter function. It is a precursor to 5-hydroxy-tryophan and serotonin, one of the neurotransmitters controlling sleep and mood. Tryptophan is not richly supplied in the diet and is considered a limiting amino acid. Tryptophan competes with leucine, isoleucine, tyrosine, phenylalanine, valine and threonine for uptake.
>
> **VALINE** is mainly utilized by muscle and brain for the formation of alanine.

- Because the bowel plays a critical role in the health of the immune system, if the bowel is being taxed, the immune system is compromised. How this works is that healthy bacteria in the bowel naturally suppress disease-causing infections. That healthy bacteria in the bowel can be destroyed by using antibiotics, eating too many processed foods with chemicals and preservatives, and poor digestion. Once this healthy bacteria is destroyed, the bowel no longer acts as a barrier to disease and leads to the immune system being compromised. This has long-term implications for diseases affecting the mind and body. (See *Chapter 9* for further discussion of the immune system.)

# Food is not enough

When you ask most people who are concerned about nutrition whether or not they have a healthy diet, the majority will answer "yes." Yet we know that the average diet is 40% fat, it is calcium-deficient and it is lacking in sufficient servings of fruit and vegetables for essential nutrients. Added to this is the diminished nutritional status of the foods we consume.

Consider:

- micronutrients are essential for the formation of the bowel,
- presence of antibiotics and preservatives in the food which can disrupt the healthy bowel bacteria,
- processing so food is prized for its convenience not its rich nutritional content.

The result is that most people are lacking the very source of health – a good diet composed of high-quality nutrients. It's as if the gas we put in our car for a trip is watered down and full of dangerous additives. It's going to be a bumpy ride, especially so if the roads are in poor shape or we encounter stormy weather conditions.

The conditions necessary in our bodies for healthy digestion and absorption include enzymes and healthy bacteria (up to three pounds of healthy gut bacteria are required in an adult), the very organisms killed by antibiotics. Think of the bowel as

## Non-essential amino acids

(can be manufactured in body as well as derived from food):

**ALANINE** aids in the metabolism of glucose. In conditions such as hypoglycemia, alanine may be used to produce glucose in order to stabilize blood levels.

**ASPARTIC ACID** performs an important role in the urea cycle where it assists in the removal of ammonia from the body. Aspartic acid can be formed from oxaloacetate in a vitamin B6-dependent reaction.

**CYSTATHIONINE** is an intermediate in the conversion of methionine to cysteine (see the SAM cycle in *Chapter 12: One Mother's Story*). Vitamin B6 is a cofactor for this reaction.

a lawn with a carpet of essential organisms. If you apply weed killer (antibiotics) to the lawn, you not only kill weeds, you also eliminate some of the healthy grass (bacteria). Without enough grass to stop them, the weeds grow back more aggressively, becoming stronger in the process. The lawn's best defense against weeds is a sufficient carpet of grass nurtured with organic compost, much like the healthy bacteria in the bowel is the body's best defense against intestinal disorders and malabsorption.

Nutrients are absorbed into the bloodstream and carried to the body's tissues through the lining of the small intestine. Even where food has been digested, malabsorption can occur from damage to these intestinal walls. This can result from disorders such as celiac disease or lactose intolerance, but can also occur because of chronic constipation or diarrhea. Malabsorption will cause nutritional deficiencies whether or not you have a good diet.

Without sufficient nutrients working together, health and vitality are compromised, illness takes hold and a compromised immune system that results has implications for future long-term diseases.

## Non-essential amino acids cont.

**CYSTEINE** and **CYSTINE** in metabolic terms, can be thought of as the same. Cystine is an oxidized form of cysteine and the body is capable of converting one to the other as required. Cysteine is a sulfur-rich amino acid, obtaining its sulfur groups from methionine. Vitamin B6 serves as a cofactor for this process. Cysteine is used in the formation of a number of essential compounds including coenzyme A, heparin, biotin, lipoic acid, glutathione, insulin and the glucose tolerance factor.

**GLUTAMINE** and **GLUTAMIC ACID** play important roles in the metabolism of urinary ammonia. Glutamic acid does not pass the blood-brain barrier but glutamine does, after which it is converted back to glutamic acid. Glutamic acid is a major excitatory neurotransmitter in the brain and spinal cord, and is the precursor of GABA, which is an inhibitory neurotransmitter.

# Problems in Down Syndrome
## The problems we all face – and a few more

When we look at digestion and absorption problems in children with Down Syndrome, we see a reflection of what's happening in the overall population, with some additional problems related to this genetic disorder. Down Syndrome is a genetic alteration that results in a change in biochemistry. The extra copy of the 21st chromosome can affect every system in the body.

## The human factory

How does that genetic alteration affect the body? It's like a factory where the chromosomes are the workers, each with his own work station. As the first worker makes the sleeve, he passes it on to the next worker who makes the lapels then passes it on to the next worker and so on. If one of the workers is working 50% faster (because that worker chromosome has three chromosomes instead of the usual two), everything in the assembly system is affected. Worker 21 is consuming more material and at a faster rate, creating deficits and excesses.

## Non-essential amino acids cont.

**GLYCINE** is a major part of the pool of amino acids which are available for the synthesis of non-essential amino acids. Glycine is readily converted into serine. Glycine is utilized in liver detoxification compounds, such as glutathione, is essential for the biosynthesis of nucleic and bile acids and is a methyl group carrier for the SAM cycle (see *Chapter 12* for more on the SAM cycle).

**ORNITHINE** participates in the formation of urea in the liver, is the precursor of amino acids such as citrulline, glutamic acid, and proline, and is used for polyamine synthesis.

**SERINE** is very reactive in the body, taking part in pyrimidine, purine, creatine and porphyrin biosynthesis. Serine takes part in a reaction with homocysteine to form cysteine. Serine is a constituent of phospholipids and is a precursor of ethanolamine and choline. Therefore serine is needed for maintaining a healthy immune system, for the proper metabolism of fats and for muscle growth.

Digestive problems for children with Down Syndrome begin at the beginning, with chewing and swallowing. Dental and related problems that occur frequently in children with Down Syndrome include:

- missing teeth and delayed eruption of teeth;
- reduced saliva;
- facial features that affect chewing and swallowing;
- enlarged tongue;
- greater incidence of gum disease and early tooth loss.

The effects of some or all of these conditions on the initial breakdown of food can be profound.

Other problems occur along the way as well.

- High rates of upper respiratory infections lead to greater use of antibiotics in children with Down Syndrome, even where it is useless for conditions such as bronchitis. As already discussed, these drugs kill off the very bacteria needed for the digestive system to function.

- In children with Down Syndrome, the bowel matures more slowly. Weaning and introduction of solid foods before the bowel is ready places stress on the digestive system.

- Greater rates of obesity in Down Syndrome are often treated with weight-loss diets producing insufficient fat for proper functioning of the gall bladder.

Research claiming to prove there is no malabsorption problem in

## Non-essential amino acids cont.

**TAURINE** is a sulfur-containing amino acid that is synthesized from methionine and cysteine, primarily in the liver with the assistance of vitamin B6. Taurine functions with glycine and GABA, two neuroinhibitory transmitters. Taurine also functions to maintain the correct composition of bile and in maintaining the solubility of cholesterol.

**TYROSINE** is a precursor to thyroid hormones and to dopa, dopamine, norepinephrine and epinephrine. Tyrosine is formed from the essential amino acid phenylalanine. Tyrosine degradation is dependent on ascorbic acid.

children with Down Syndrome ignores the evidence: those with Down Syndrome have higher than normal rates of chronic constipation, diarrhea, celiac disease and gluten intolerance.[2, 3, 4]

## The Autism bowel connection

And that's not all: children with Down Syndrome are 20 times more likely than those in the general population to have Autism, a disease that is increasing in the overall population of children.[5, 6] Research now points to a definite connection between Autism and bowel problems.

Autism is what is known as a spectrum disorder: numerous symptoms, most notably in communication and social interaction, can exist in a wide range of combinations and severity. Autism is not present at birth, but develops during the first three years of a child's life. Recent research has indicated a link between Autism and bowel disorders, especially gluten and lactose intolerance.

What's the connection? There is evidence showing that people with Autism are unable to break down a protein in milk. Morphine-like compounds are produced as a result which find their way to the brain, causing cell dysfunction. The most profound effect on symptoms of Autism comes from removing milk and gluten from the bowel.[7] Some process affecting the bowel, such as infection, causes the

**DEFINING MOMENT**

**Protein:**
A macronutrient, like fat and carbohydrates, that provides energy for the body. Proteins are digested in the gastrointestinal tract and broken down into amino acids. The amino acids are then used to form new proteins in the body. Protein-rich substances in our body include muscle, blood, ligaments, skin, internal organs, glands, nails and hair. Enzymes, hormones and antibodies are also composed of protein.

**Chromosomes:**
The genetic material present in cells is in the form of chromosomes. Human cells have 46 chromosomes in two sets of 23 pairs. Genes are portions of chromosomes.

**Down Syndrome and Vitamin Therapy**

digestion of certain proteins to become abnormal. Recent research indicates that these proteins affect the brain, becoming toxic to the brain (neuro-toxic) and resulting in the damage associated with Autism. This explains why we see the onset of Autism most commonly around the age of two, not at birth. (For more information on Autism, see *Chapter 4*.)

## Solutions

### It all comes back to synergy

It almost goes without saying that when we talk about nutritional status, we look first to the raw material: food. It's important to remember the law of synergy – nutrients don't work in isolation. This means that the diet must be complete so that nutrients which serve as co-factors or catalysts for others are present and in sufficient quality and quantity. For example, vitamin E and zinc are required for proper vitamin A metabolism; riboflavin (vitamin B2) helps convert vitamin B6 into other metabolic forms; vitamin D increases calcium absorption.

But in today's world, it isn't always feasible to get all of our nutritional needs met with food.

### DEFINING MOMENT

**Hormones:**
Biological substances made up of proteins and used to regulate body functions such as growth and metabolism.

**Metabolism:**
Chemical reactions that take place in the cells of the body; includes breakdown of organic compounds to yield energy (catabolism) and synthesis of materials from simpler substances (anabolism).

### DEFINING MOMENT

**Enzymes:**
Also referred to as the "sparks of life." These biological substances are made up of proteins and act as catalysts. They are essential for digesting food, stimulating the brain, providing cellular energy and repairing all tissues, organs and cells.

We look to nutritional supplementation because:

- the diet is missing certain nutrients,
- the nutrients are of poor quality due to food production methods,
- and/or there is a digestive problem causing malabsorption of nutrients.

## DEFINING MOMENT

### Bowel:
The gastrointestinal system of the body extending from the stomach to the anal opening. Includes small intestine (composed of the duodenum, jejunum, and ileum) and colon (large intestine).

## Five keys to healthy digestion
The essential factors in ensuring that your body gets what it needs from food and nutritional supplements are:

- nutrients available in sufficient quantities and combinations;
- digestion aided by enzymes and healthy bacteria;
- adequate absorption of nutrients for use by the body;
- proper metabolism where food is efficiently converted into energy;
- healthy elimination of waste, essential in avoiding toxicity.

## Treat the illness
One of the biggest stumbling blocks to use of nutritional supplements for children with Down Syndrome is an unwillingness to treat the digestive-related illness separately from the Down Syndrome. In the case of malabsorption and Down Syndrome, critics argue against the use of nutritional therapy unless we can prove that the digestive disorder is related to the genetic condition. The result of this faulty logic is a conclusion that says it's fine to provide nutritional treatment we know is safe and effective for malabsorption problems in the general population, but not for individuals with Down Syndrome. This amounts to an unethical withholding of treatment simply because of the presence of Down Syndrome.

We know that missing nutrients and malabsorption cause a chain reaction of problems in the body. We know that digestion and absorption are essential for health and that these are often compromised by a variety of causes. We have growing rates of illness and disease. And we know that nutritional therapy can correct these deficiencies and imbalances, improving health and preventing disease, without causing harm.

## Solve the problem

It isn't necessary to prove a link between Down Syndrome and malabsorption in order to treat problems in the bowel. If we accept that we must "solve the problem" with or without regard to any Down Syndrome connection, we follow the accepted route for any nutritional therapy:

- investigate the symptoms;
- assess any blood or other lab reports;
- remove any sources of allergy or intolerance;
- restore fibre, digestive enzymes and healthy bacteria;

### Are you eating antibiotics?

I recently attended a lecture where the audience was asked who had taken an antibiotic during the previous week. Only one person indicated they had. The lecturer then asked how many people had eaten chicken or beef during the previous week. Virtually everyone in the audience replied that they had. The lecturer then told the audience that they had all had antibiotics the previous week, since these drugs are routinely fed to chickens and cows to increase growth and yield and prevent mastitis.

- give probiotics such as acidophilus and bifidus instead of, or in addition to, antibiotics to increase the beneficial intestinal flora essential for proper digestion;
- supplement missing or insufficient nutrients;
- monitor the progress;
- and above all, do no harm.

## Testing for Celiac Disease

While several diagnostic tests exist for diagnosis of Celiac Disease, the gold standard of testing is the small bowel biopsy. This is an invasive procedure requiring anaesthetic. Because of the heightened sensitivity to anaesthetic in children with Down Syndrome, parents should be cautious in allowing this method of diagnosis for Celiac Disease, using less invasive methods such as tTG before moving to this biopsy.

The tTG test is a specific and highly effective method for diagnosing Celiac Disease with almost 100% accuracy.[8, 9] This test is a blood test which measures the antibodies to the enzymes responsible for breaking down gluten. You have to be on gluten products while taking this test and the results should be interpreted by a doctor who is experienced in this area. The tTG test allows you to avoid the invasive biopsy with its inherent risk from anesthetic.

From the time of the first presentation of symptoms of Celiac Disease, patients average 10 years before the cause is diagnosed correctly. In Japan, where the use of the tTG test is widespread, the average time between presentation

## Celiac Disease: the malabsorption problem

Commonly known as gluten intolerance, Celiac Disease happens when the lining of the small intestine becomes damaged from exposure to gluten (a rye and wheat protein). It results in malabsorption of nutrients with accompanying failure to grow and thrive. Constipation and diarrhea are common, as well as abdominal distention, large bulky stools and irritability. While early diagnosis is important and will result in the removal of gluten from the diet, it won't change the presence of Celiac Disease. This means that the absorption portion of the bowel (called the villi) is destroyed and it is absolutely essential to give the bowel good support with lots of water, fibre, acidophilus and enzymes.

## Lactose intolerance

There is an increased incidence of lactose intolerance in Down Syndrome. The symptoms mimic those of gluten intolerance: gas, bloating, diarrhea. Therefore, it is important to conduct a tTG test (see above) to determine whether or not the origin of the problem is gluten.

of symptoms and diagnosis is six months. This provides ample proof of the value of the test.

# Fibre-rich foods

| | SERVING SIZE | TOTAL FIBRE (GRAMS) |
|---|---|---|
| **FIBRE-RICH GRAINS** | | |
| Barley | 1/2 cup | 15.60 |
| All-Bran Buds with Psyllium | 1/3 cup | 12.7 |
| Psyllium fibre supplement | up to 3 tsp/day | up to 9.0 |
| Bran | 1 ounce | 8.72 |
| Rice, brown | 1/2 cup | 5.27 |
| Lentils | 1/2 cup | 5.22 |
| Oat bran | 1 ounce | 4.08 |
| Wheat germ | 1 ounce | 4.05 |
| Oatmeal | 1 ounce | 2.51 |
| Whole wheat bread | 1 slice | 2.11 |
| **FIBRE-RICH VEGETABLES AND LEGUMES** | | |
| Kidney beans | 1/2 cup | 5.48 |
| Brown beans | 1/2 cup | 4.64 |
| Almonds, roasted | 1/4 cup | 3.98 |
| Artichoke | 1 globe | 3.96 |
| Green peas | 1/2 cup | 3.52 |
| Peanuts, roasted | 1/4 cup | 3.17 |
| Corn | 1/2 cup | 3.03 |
| Broccoli | 1/2 cup | 2.58 |
| Carrots | 1/2 cup | 2.42 |
| Cauliflower | 1/2 cup | 2.30 |
| Spinach | 1/2 cup | 2.07 |
| Potato, baked w/skin | 1/2 cup | 1.95 |
| **FIBRE-RICH FRUIT** | | |
| Prunes, canned | 1/2 cup | 6.88 |
| Pear, with peel | 1 medium | 4.32 |
| Blackberries | 1/2 cup | 3.72 |
| Grapefruit | 1 medium | 3.61 |
| Raspberries | 1/2 cup | 3.15 |
| Orange | 1 medium | 3.14 |
| Apple with peel | 1 medium | 2.76 |
| Banana | 1 medium | 2.19 |

# Closing comments from Kent:

*I was recently consulted by a pediatrician on what to do about "functional constipation." I asked her what she meant by this term and she replied that "It is just constant constipation for which you don't know the cause." I asked her if she used in her medical practice good blends of soluble and insoluble fibres, enzymes and acidophilus – the substances that make up the bulk of human fecal matter. Her answer: "No, I only give the symptomatic relievers (ie. laxatives)." I suggested she try giving the fundamental components of the bowel (water, fibre, acidophilus and enzymes). She called me later expressing her absolute amazement that this protocol worked and her patient was now doing very well.*

*I have generally found that children with Down Syndrome who have problems with digestion need more involved consultation on an individual basis. This is a list of things that must be considered:*

1. *Medical conditions diagnosed by a doctor, for instance, a genetic abnormality, or a subsequent drug condition whereby, for example, the bowel may need drug therapy to suppress acid. This therapy may interfere with digestion and the absorption of food and key nutrients.*

2. *Celiac Disease, which should be screened for with a tTG test.*

3. *Food allergies, which can be tested for with blood tests and elimination diets.*

4. *General bowel support with the correct amounts of enzymes, probiotics and fibre. – K.M.*

# Endnotes

1. Horvath, K., et al. (1999) "Gastrointestinal abnormalities in children with autistic disorder." *Journal of Pediatrics* 135(5): 559-93.

2. Zachor, D.A., (2000) "Down syndrome and Celiac Disease: A Review." *Down Syndrome Quarterly* 5(4): 1-5.

3. Mackey, J., et al. (2001) "Frequency of celiac disease in individuals with Down syndrome in the United States." *Clinical Pediatrics* (Philadelphia). 40(5): 249-52.

4. Book, L., et al. (2001) "Prevalence and clinical characteristics of celiac disease in Downs syndrome in a US study." *American Journal of Medical Genetics.* 98(1): 70-4.

5. Kent, L., et al. (1999) "Comorbidity of autistic spectrum disorders in children with Down syndrome." *Developmental Medicine and Child Neurology* 41(3): 153-8

6. Kapell, D., et al. (1998) "Prevalence of chronic medical conditions in adults with mental retardation: comparison with the general population." *Mental Retardation* 36(4): 269-79.

7. Reichelt, K-L., et al. (1990) "Gluten, milk proteins and autism: dietary intervention effects on behavior and peptide secretion." *Journal of Applied Nutrition* 42:1-8.

8. Reeves, G.E., et al. (2000) "The measurement of IgA and IgG transglutaminase antibodies in celiac disease: a comparison with current diagnostic methods." *Pathology.* 32(3):181-5.

9. Csizmadia, C.G., et al. (2000) "Accuracy and cost-effectiveness of a new strategy to screen for celiac disease in children with Down syndrome." *Journal of Pediatrics.* 137(6): 756-61. psychomotor development. Archives of Disease in Childhood. 80(4):334-8.

# AUSTIN'S STORY

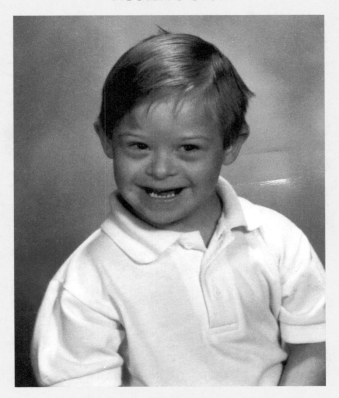

Ellen Abshire says she can't say what effect vitamins have had on her six-year-old son, Austin, since he's been on MSB almost his entire life. What she does know for sure is that he's a healthy, active little boy and that "everyone just loves Austin."

Austin has been on MSB vitamins since he was nine months old and his mother describes him as "high-functioning and in good health. His muscle tone is great, he's solid as a rock. And he can handle a computer like an adult."

Ellen heard about vitamin supplements for children with Down Syndrome from her pediatrician's nurse, and from her mother who had seen a television program on the subject. But it was a conversation with another mother whose son had problems that were helped by Nutri-Chem's MSB formula that got her started. Aside from keeping Austin healthy now, Ellen's main goal is to prevent future brain deterioration from oxidative stress.

"My goal for Austin is that he grow up healthy and some day have a real job, not something where he's paid 25 cents an hour. He's such a character, I think he could be an actor some day."

# FREE RADICALS AND OXIDATIVE STRESS

*SOME TIME AGO, I WAS PREPARING A TALK to parents about oxidative stress and free radicals. I was struggling with how best to describe this phenomenon when my then-11-year-old son, Andrew, flew across the carpet. "Hey Dad, shake my hand!" he called, reaching out to touch me. As he did so, a spark flew. Andrew had just become a free radical. In biological systems, he would represent trouble. Fortunately for our household, I stopped the free-floating spark when I took Andrew's hand, stopping the spark's chain reaction. I had become Andrew's antioxidant. – K.M.*

## WHAT WILL I LEARN?

▸ How free radicals damage cells.

▸ Why oxidative stress is more harmful to people with Down Syndrome.

▸ How antioxidants can help stop the damage.

If you're old enough to remember the computer craze Pac Man, you have an idea about free radicals and what they can do. In the game, the wild little Pac Man creature zoomed around, creating havoc by gobbling up anything in its path. Difficult to catch because of his speed and ability to hit his target, he was chased and finally destroyed by his enemy, the ghosts.

Free radicals are the Pac Men inside your body. These highly reactive molecules contain an unpaired electron. They roam around freely, looking for a mate: an unmatched electron to which they can attach. You might think of them as unstable fellows looking for trouble, because when they find what they're looking for these biological bad boys cause serious damage to cells and genetic material.

## Where do they come from?

You already have free radicals inside your body in small numbers. They occur naturally from the oxygen of the air we breathe and from biochemical processes within our bodies. When they don't get out of control free radicals actually perform a number of vital tasks. Some are found in the immune system's white blood cells, blasting bacteria just like our body's own radiation system. Others work on producing energy through creation of hormones and enzymes. In the right circumstances, your body uses its own enzymes to keep free radicals under control. These include superoxide dismutase (SOD), catalase and glutathione peroxidase.

## Introducing free radicals

It's not one size fits all when it comes to free radicals. There are different types, each with its own composition and moniker. These are: superoxide, hydroxy radicals, hydrogen peroxide, lipid peroxides, hypochlorite radicals, nitric oxide, singlet oxygen. Some are more powerful than others, and each may have its own preferred target.

## How do things go wrong?

Just like Pac Man, free radicals can get out of control. It happens from exposure to chemicals, the sun or from a breakdown or imbalance in the body's own processes. When this happens, there's a multiplying effect. Remember that the free radical is an unpaired, unstable molecule looking for an electron mate. As it does so it becomes highly charged, sucking up electrons from other molecules, turning them into free radicals. They repeat the process which creates other free radicals and so on. The result is oxidation, a process that destroys cells, tissues and genetic material in your body. To see the effects of oxidation, look at what happens to an apple you cut in half and leave on the counter. The exposed flesh turns brown, then rots. Such is the power of oxidation.

In humans, oxidative stress from an excess of free radicals is implicated in conditions we typically associate with aging: memory loss, Alzheimer's, heart disease and cancer.[1] Free radicals can damage cells and the genetic material stored inside them. The brain is particularly vulnerable to free radicals because of its structure and function. It has very little of the defensive enzyme catalase.

**DEFINING MOMENT**

**HYDROGEN:** Key component of many biological/organic molecules in our bodies; can also be a very powerful free radical.

**OXYGEN:** Required for breathing; essential element that is a key component of many biological/organic molecules in our bodies; extremely chemically active

**OXIDATION:** When an atom or molecule loses electrons, it is oxidized; (i.e. when an antioxidant steals an electron from a fat, the fat has been oxidized).

**POLYUNSATURATED:** Fats saturated with two or more hydrogen atoms.

It has a high polyunsaturated fat content and also a high oxygen requirement (which could indirectly cause free radicals).

## Do people with Down Syndrome experience more oxidative stress?

How do we know there is oxidative stress in children with Down Syndrome? One of the most important pieces of evidence noted in reviewing lab reports is the disease pattern found in individuals with Down Syndrome. This disease pattern is similar to that of diseases associated with oxidative stress found in the non-Down Syndrome population. These include: weakened immune system (or altered or disturbed immune system), Alzheimer's disease, leukemia and cataracts.

At Nutri-Chem when we analyze blood tests of children with Down Syndrome, we find that in over 70% of cases the levels of antioxidant vitamins E, A, and coenzyme Q10 are deficient. (We are using ranges which reflect the so-called "normal" population, which is itself generally nutritionally deficient.)

In other genetic defects there is often a missing piece or a miscoding of information. In Down Syndrome, the coding is perfect, there's simply an extra perfect chromosome. This has resulted in the theory of gene over-dosage with a resulting over-expression of certain enzymes.[2, 3, 4, 5]

The gene for superoxide dismutase (SOD), one of the enzymes that controls free radicals, is found on the 21st chromosome.

# Interrelationships between free radicals and antioxidants

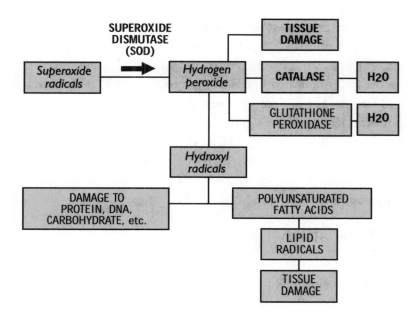

Antioxidant Enzymes: SOD, Glutathione, peroxidase, and catalase act to assist the breakdown of free radicals.

Dietary Antioxidants: vitamin E, vitamin C, lipoic acid, etc., act to quench free radicals and inhibit damage to tissues and biological molecules.

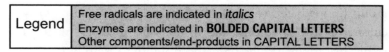

| Legend | Free radicals are indicated in *italics* |
| | Enzymes are indicated in **BOLDED CAPITAL LETTERS** |
| | Other components/end-products in CAPITAL LETTERS |

Source: Free Radical Biology and Medicine (1996) 20(5) 679

In normal metabolism, superoxide is dismutased or changed into hydrogen peroxide. This is then converted by glutathione peroxidase or catalase into harmless water. In Down Syndrome there is excess SOD and a normal genetic complement of glutathione peroxidase and catalase. This results in an excess production of hydrogen peroxide which, when not converted to water, turns into a free radical (hydroxyl radical). This is one of the radicals implicated in damage to protein, DNA, carbohydrate and fats. (In fact, it's the most reactive radical, and therefore very powerful.) The greatest significance for this is found in the brain. By the age of 35, the brain of a person with Down Syndrome resembles that of someone with Alzheimer's disease, showing similar plaques and lesions.[6, 7, 8] (See *Chapter 10* for more information on the brain.)

## Nature study

The best-known in vitro study (i.e. done in test tubes) on the potential of antioxidants to prevent brain cell death (apoptosis), was the *Nature* study done by Buscaglio and Yanker.[9]

In this study, the researchers cultured brain cells from individuals with Down Syndrome in test tubes. After two weeks they found that 60% of the brain cells had spontaneously died through a process called apoptosis. Brain cells from the control group (individuals who did NOT have Down Syndrome) were cultured at the same time and in the same growing media. The result was dramatically different from the group with Down Syndrome: no brain cells died from the control group. In fact, they had more than 100% of the brain cells which meant that the brain cells in the non-Down Syndrome group actually grew in this environment over a two-week period.

Buscaglio, et al then repeated this same experiment. However, this time vitamin E and other antioxidants were added to the test tubes of the Down Syndrome brain cells. The result was that 100% of the Down Syndrome brain cells were now alive after two weeks. This meant that the vitamin E and other antioxidants had kept the Down Syndrome brain cells alive compared to the experiment without antioxidants where 60% of the Down Syndrome cells died.

## ICMT study

On the heels of the Buscaglio and Yanker *Nature* study (see above), Nutri-Chem scientists realized that there was not yet "in vivo" (or living) evidence of oxidative stress in individuals with Down Syndrome. Therefore, in 1998 Nutri-Chem's International Center for Metabolic Testing undertook a study aimed at documenting the levels of oxidative stress in children with Down Syndrome as compared to children without the genetic disorder.

There was a good deal of research showing that antioxidants could benefit diseases where oxidative stress was present. And there was in vitro evidence of oxidative stress in Down Syndrome from Buscaglio and Yanker's study. However, we believed that to provide a stronger case for antioxidant supplementation in Down Syndrome, we needed direct evidence of oxidative stress in vivo, in living children. This was the reason that Nutri-Chem's International Centre for Metabolic Testing undertook our 1998 study. The purpose was to document levels of oxidative stress in children with and without Down Syndrome.

We studied urine samples from 166 participants comprised of children with Down Syndrome and their siblings. They ranged in age from 2 to 11. We investigated the level of 8-hydroxy-2'deoxyguanosine (8oHdG), a biomarker of DNA damage, and found it elevated in the children with Down Syndrome as compared to their siblings.[10] This showed elevated oxidative stress in Down Syndrome since DNA damage reflects increased degenerative processes. This data was consistent with the observed premature aging, increased incidence of cataracts and early Alzheimer-like changes in people with Down Syndrome.

Our study also looked at damage to lipids/fats in the urine. Here too we saw elevations of oxidative damage to an established marker called TBARS (thiobarbituric acid reactive substances).

Taken together, the results provide a strong case for the presence of oxidative stress in children with Down Syndrome.

## The case for vitamin E

Vitamin E's main function is to reduce oxidative damage to fats and lipids. When given vitamin E, there is a noted reduction of oxidative damage in individuals with Down Syndrome.

### Vitamin E: Natural versus Synthetic

Dr. Keith Ingold proved that synthetic vitamin E is selectively destroyed by the liver rendering the synthetic vitamin E useless.[13] You can tell which vitamin E you are purchasing by reading the label closely. Synthetic vitamin E has an "L" in its description called dl alpha-tocopherol. Natural vitamin E has no "L" and is called -D-alphatocopherol. Hence the phrase "to hell with the L"!

Vitamin E has proven to reduce apoptosis (cell death) in test tubes, reduce lipid damage "in vivo" of children with Down Syndrome and to be depressed in the blood of children with Down Syndrome. In the general population, vitamin E has proven to improve dramatically the outcome of Alzheimer's disease and to improve the immune system by as much as seven times.[11, 12] It is proven to be safe with a history of over 90 years of usage. Vitamin E has NOT been used nor recommended by the medical establishment for individuals with Down Syndrome despite the substantial amount of evidence regarding its safety and benefit.

Other forms of tocopherol such as Gamma-tocopherol may have benefit as well and should be included in supplements because Gamma-tocopherol quenches the nitroso free radical which can be particularly dangerous in the brain.[14]

# Radical solutions

Just as with the ghosts that zapped Pac Man, antioxidants are the enemy of excessive free radicals. They bind to electrons and deprive the biochemical bad boys of their chance to pull electrons from other cells. Without the possibility of an attachment, the free radical moves on, eventually running out of options and dying. In fact, while they do burn hot, free radicals don't burn for long because they have a short lifespan. This stops the cascading chain reaction where free radicals reproduce themselves.

After analyzing countless lab reports we have noted a host of other antioxidants which are depressed in individuals with Down Syndrome and that are just as essential as vitamin E. They are vitamin A, vitamin C, selenium and co-enzyme Q10. However if vitamin E is not used with its overwhelming evidence of benefit, what hope do we have of having the medical establishment using these other essential antioxidants in individuals with Down Syndrome.

Laboratory testing of your child for these levels (discussed in *Chapter 11* on lab testing) provides parents and their physicians the lab evidence for supplementing these essential antioxidants with confidence just as they would supplement iron to their child after a lab test shows depressed iron levels.

Nutrients supply these valuable antioxidants. The most commonly-used and studied antioxidants are vitamins A, C and E, beta-carotene, selenium and co-enzyme Q10. In addition to beta-carotene, other carotenoids, such as lycopene, alpha-carotene and lutein are also antioxidants. Cysteine, an amino acid necessary for glutathione, and glutathione itself, are antioxidants. Lipoic acid helps to recycle vitamins C, E and glutathione.

In addition to these key antioxidants which have direct impact on free radical activity, there is a host of antioxidant support systems in the body that require complete nutritional support. This means you need proper protein, correct fats and oils, correct minerals, lots of carotenoids found in coloured fruits and vegetables and the proper micronutrients.

Ideally, you should have your child tested for levels of antioxidants and markers of lipid peroxidation. This would include tests for indirect and direct functional tests for antioxidants (explained in *Chapter 11* in the section on lab testing).

## How much of a good thing is enough?

The amount of antioxidants needed is related to the level of free radicals and oxidative stress. The more free radicals, the more antioxidants are needed. Multiple antioxidants must be used, because they interact. Antioxidant defense is like a table top balanced on legs. If one leg is too short, the whole table tips over.

In your car, a faulty engine creates problems – sparks, debris and soot. In your body, it's oxidation that makes things dirty and antioxidants that clean up the dirt. But what about the dirty rags that are left behind? Lipoic acid is the detergent that washes up this biological dirty laundry, getting right inside the engine of your cells (the mitachondria).

**Down Syndrome and Vitamin Therapy**

# Closing comments from Kent:

*Parents need to be aware that one of the problems with nutritional pharmacology is the tendency of professionals to want to use vitamins in the same fashion as others use drugs. This approach is derived from a drug model that relies on high doses of a single source. Too many nutritional scientists want to use this model for evidence that will support vitamin supplements. The problem with this approach is that our basic biology and biochemistry teaches us that we need ALL of the antioxidants together in a balanced format to give us good results with safe use. Think of the table legs that support the table: you can't use one leg only or the table will not stand. Similarly, you need a good combination of antioxidants to help support your child's health.*

*I would advise parents have testing done to measure your child's key antioxidants, and give these nutrients in a balanced multinutrient combination. Remember that there is a great deal of evidence for the benefits of using antioxidants in Down Syndrome, especially vitamin E. And also remember that the medical establishment is waiting for evidence that utilizes an inappropriate drug model to prove the efficacy of vitamin supplements.*
*– K.M.*

# Endnotes

1. Kehrer, J.P., and Smith, C.V. (1994) "Free radicals in biology: sources, reactivities, and roles in the etiology of human diseases." *Natural Antioxidants in Health and Disease* (Ed. Frei, B) Academic Press p 25-64

2. Feaster, W.W., et al. (1977) "Dosage effects for superoxide dismutase in nucleated cells aneuploid for chromosome 21." *American Journal of Human Genetics* 29: 563-570.

3. Sinet, P.M., et al. (1975) "Superoxide dismutase activities of blood platelets in trisomy 21." *Biochemical and Biophysical Research Communications* 67: 904-909.

4. Sinet, P-M., et al. (1976) "Trisomie 21 et superoxyde dismutase-1 (IPO-A)" *Experimental Cell Research* 97: 47-55.

5. Sinet, P.M. (1982) "Metabolism of oxygen derivatives in Down's syndrome." *Annals of the New York Academy of Science* 396: 83-94.

6. Wisniewski, H.M. and Rabe, A. (1985) "Discrepancy between Alzheimer-type neuropathology and dementia in persons with Down's syndrome." *Annals of the New York Academy of Science* 477: 247-260.

7. Rabe, A., et al. (1990) *Relationship of Down's syndrome to Alzheimer's disease. Application of Basic Neuroscience to Child Psychiatry* (eds. Deutsch, S.I., Weizman, A. and Weizman, R., Plenum Press, New York) pp 325-340.

8. Kolata, G. (1985) "Down-syndrome-Alzheimer's linked." *Science* 230: 1152-1153.

9. Buscaglio, J., and Yanker, B.A. (1995) "Apoptosis and increased generation of reactive oxygen species in Down's syndrome neurons in vitro." *Nature* 378: 776-779

10. Jovanovic, S., et al. (1998) "Biomarkers of oxidative stress are significantly elevated in Down syndrome." *Free Radical Biology and Medicine* 25: 1044-48.

11. Sano, M., et al. (1997) "A controlled trial of selegiline, alpha-tocopherol, or both as treatment for Alzheimer's disease." *New England Journal of Medicine* 336: 1216-22.

12. Meydani, S., et al. (1997) "Vitamin E supplementation and in vivo immune response in healthy elderly subjects." *Journal of the American Medical Association* 277: 1380-86.

13. Burton, G.W., et al. (1998). "Human plasma and tissue alpha-tocopherol concentrations in response to supplementation with deuterated natural and synthetic vitamin E." *American Journal of Clinical Nutrition* 67: 669-684.

14. Christen, S., et al (1997) "Gamma-tocopherol traps mutagenic electrophiles such as Nox and complements alpha-tocopherol: physiological implications." *Proceedings of the National Academy of Sciences U.S.A.* 94: 3217-3222.

# KAILIN'S STORY

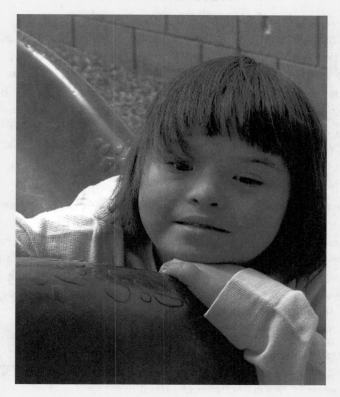

For parents, having a child with Down Syndrome changes their lives. For Mary Bryant, it also brought a career change. Living in Nevada, Mary was an executive in the high-pressure gaming industry. "I was 39 when Kailin was born. My job was day and night, 60 to 70 hours a week. It was not a very forgiving industry." Now, Mary works as associate director of a local disability organization. It's a shift that mirrors Mary's own shift in attitude about her daughter who was born with Down Syndrome.

"When Kailin was born, I felt there was something wrong with her. I've had a real attitude change since then. Now I look at Kailin as just different, and perfect the way she is."

Kailin has been on MSB since infancy. She's had metabolic testing done at Nutri-Chem, and receives a customized formula. "It improves her brain function and her health. Kailin has a really poor diet. She doesn't understand that fast foods are bad and she really likes them. So MSB ensures that she has an adequate supply of nutrients," Mary says.

"Basically, Kailin is very healthy, She has had significant sinus infections and has been on antibiotics a lot, but we're trying now to go without antibiotics because we know that Kailin's sinus cavities are growing. She has not had any ear infections but has had some constipation which is getting better. Kailin does have a lot of allergies especially to wheat and dairy. We took her off both for a while, but it was torture for her. We found she was sneaking those foods."

This independent stance is serving Kailin well in other areas, however. She's an outgoing little girl who is very active at her day care and school where she's known as "KK" to her friends. She's become a six-year-old yoga wonder – her yoga teacher calls her "yoga-adept." Kailin is now acting as a yoga teaching assistant at the pre-school she and her sister attend. She's demonstrating yoga poses and helping the other children with theirs. This summer, she will continue her yoga teaching assistant role when she attends camp.

Kailin's mother says her health and development is the result of many things including her relationship with younger sister, Eilish, and being in the mainstream of school life. She has stayed on MSB throughout, and also takes piracetam. Mary says she has stuck with Nutri-Chem because of its track record with children with Down Syndrome, its research and testing experience, and the quality of its formula.

"Our whole family is now on vitamins. Having Kailin improved our lives in a great way," Mary says. "We know that people with Down Syndrome tend to be overweight and somewhat sedentary, so we get out as a family and do lots of exercise. She's changed the way we live and greatly enriched our lives. And MSB has greatly enriched Kailin's life and is helping her to be all she can be."

# CHAPTER 9

# THE IMMUNE AND THYROID SYSTEMS

*NOTHING UPSETS ME MORE than seeing the looks of resignation and defeat on the faces of parents as they listen to so-called experts outline all of the serious conditions and diseases that await their children with Down Syndrome as they grow older. What would happen if you had a room full of parents of non-Down Syndrome kids hearing nothing but doom and gloom where their children were concerned: that a certain number of their children would die of drug overdose; another percentage from car accidents due to drunk driving, and still more from suicide; or that many of their kids would fail and/or drop out of school, commit crimes and spend time in jail? Why describe all the possible problems their children might face without expressing any of the good news and positive things their kids may accomplish? Where is the sense of hope and optimism parents need to feel in order to face an uncertain future?*

## WHAT WILL I LEARN?

- How your immune system works – and why it fails.

- Why people with Down Syndrome experience more immune system problems.

- How nutrients can help.

- How the thyroid functions.

- Whether vaccinations are safe for your child.

*No health professional would treat an audience of parents in such a manner – except when it comes to parents of kids with Down Syndrome. This does a disservice to parents and contributes nothing to help prevent future problems and keep children healthy and growing despite their genetic disorder.*

*I don't understand how those who profess to be healers can be satisfied to stop at outlining potential problems without offering any solutions. Because there ARE solutions. The greatest of these is the body's own ability to heal itself, and that's where the immune system comes in. It is one of nature's most powerful and most intricate systems. When it's healthy and strong, the immune system provides the solutions, and the hope, that parents are seeking for their children.– K.M.*

## DEFINING MOMENT

**Antigen:** foreign invaders (bacteria, virus, toxin)

**Antibody (also known as immunoglobulin):** proteins produced by white blood cells that attach to antigens and disable them

**Lymph:** fluid that carries nutrients from blood to cells and returns waste from cells to blood

**White blood cells (leukocytes):** Most important part of immune system consisting of many different types of cells that destroy bacteria and viruses

**Lymphocyte:** a type of white blood cell divided into two categories: B cells which are made in the bone marrow and produce antibodies; T cells which mature in the thymus and attack invading organisms

# The healthy immune system

## A line of defense

Your immune system is a silent army of protection against disease. The soldiers do their work without you even realizing it, but if this defense system wasn't working you'd soon know it – your body would be invaded by bacteria, viruses and microbes. Yet sickness isn't the only sign of a weak immune system. Our energy and vitality (including mental alertness) depend on a strong immune system. It's also the source of healing when invasion occurs, and is now being studied for its role destroying free radicals – atoms that damage cells and tissues through oxidation and are implicated in cancers and in the aging process.

As with all systems, your immune system consists of many inter-related parts: skin, thymus, spleen, lymph system (vessels and fluid), bone marrow, white blood cells, antibodies, hormones and the complement system (a series of proteins that work with antibodies). The most significant sign of vitamin deficiency is a weak immune system because of the crucial role nutrients play in developing and maintaining this healthy army of defense.

# When it works

## Baby Steps

When you're born, your immune system system is already at work, but it's like any newborn – immature and in need of development. You aren't born with the ability to walk, but you are born with the potential. Over time, your legs develop and grow stronger, but it takes something else – experience – before you're able to walk. Just watch a baby who crawls, then turns into a toddler and storms around the house pulling knickknacks off the shelves and reaching for door handles to the outside world. It takes a few false starts and a good deal of falling down before they get it right. Babies learn to walk.

Your immune system develops as you grow, learning how to function through the experience of fighting infections and disease. With exposure to the enemy, the immune system learns to identify foreign invaders (antigens) and to produce the necessary defenses (antibodies).

At Nutri-Chem, we recommend that all children use vaccinations without thimerosal. This may be of even more

## Vaccinations and your child

Vaccinating children has been one of medicine's most beneficial actions in dramatically reducing serious childhood diseases. That being said, it has been very disturbing that the preservative thimerosal was used in many vaccines given to children less than six months of age.[1] It has been suggested that thimerosal is converted to ethyl mercury in the body, and we have no toxicity data for this form of mercury. There is concern that ethyl mercury may potentially be more neurotoxic than methyl mercury itself.

importance for children with Down Syndrome. Some researchers suggest that children with Down Syndrome are more susceptible to developing Autism (see *Chapter 4: Autism and Down Syndrome* for more on this), and there is a suggested link between Autism and vaccines with mercury content. Given this suspected link, children with Down Syndrome should not be exposed to vaccines containing thimerosal.

## Walking Tall

White blood cells are the frontline soldiers of defense in your immune system. Because of their importance, white blood cells are used as indicators of a healthy immune system. There are many different types of white blood cells in your body, and collectively they're known as leukocytes. Unlike other cells, leukocytes can act as independent, single-cell organisms that can travel around and alter other substances. Some white blood cells reproduce on their own, while others are manufactured in bone marrow.

Lymphocytes (T cells and B cells) identify and destroy the specific viruses, bacteria, fungi and cancer cells that can invade the body. They learn to recognize and remember antigens which threaten harm, and to destroy them by producing antibodies (also known as immunoglobulins). These antibodies (proteins) are Y-shaped. The tips can bind to an antigen and disable it.

White blood cells called monocytes are known as the immune system's "garbage collectors." They turn into macrophages when they leave the bone marrow where they are produced and travel through the blood system into tissue. As they move freely, monocytes collect and carry away foreign substances and damaged or aging cells, with macrophages performing the same function in tissue.

Granulocytes are the third class of leukocytes. They are divided into: neutrophils (the most common type of white blood cell) which destroy bacteria; eosinophils which destroy antigen-antibody combinations; and basophils which carry histamine to the source of infection creating inflammation which brings more blood to fight off the infection.

The lymphatic system is the other major division of the immune system's army. This set of organs, vessels and fluid provides a continuous cleansing action. The thymus, a gland located just above the breastbone, is where T cells mature. Lymph nodes, tonsils and spleen all play a role in trapping and destroying antigens. The lymph itself is a clear liquid that is really blood plasma without any red or white cells. It circulates throughout the body via lymphatic vessels, bathing cells with nutrients and returning waste to the bloodstream.

## Falling down

It's easy to see your immune system at work when a cut heals or you recover from a cold or flu. But while you may not see your immune system weakening, the evidence is there in greater susceptibility to infections and disease and slower rates of recovery. The immune system is highly interactive and its many component parts must be functioning for it to respond properly to attack. Just like you, your immune system has the ability to learn and remember. This is what enables it to differentiate between cells and organisms that are "you" and belong from those that are foreign invaders and need to be destroyed. So it's not only the immune system's ability to respond, it's also the nature of that response that determines whether or not your body has a protective army or a mutinous squadron inside. If the immune system gets it wrong, your body can literally attack itself. This is known as autoimmunity.

Your immune system learns how to perform its function with practice, each time it deals with an infection. If you suppress infections with antibiotics unnecessarily, you hinder this learning process and thus the body's ability to heal itself.

Other causes of damage to your immune system are disease, stress, environmental pollutants, poor sleep habits and drugs including antibiotics and chemotherapy. These are attacks from outside, offensive in nature. Your immune system is internal. If it responds improperly it can mutiny, becoming an enemy that attacks from within. With the right response, however, it is your system of defense.

Conventional wisdom says that as we age, our immune system ages with us. Researchers are now questioning this commonly-held view and looking at whether we've got it all wrong – it's really a weak immune system that creates the symptoms normally associated with aging. This is related to a process called oxidation which creates an excess of free radicals. These unstable and highly reactive molecules can damage cells and genetic material and weaken DNA, protein or fat.

## The immune system and Down Syndrome

Immune dysfunction is a classic characteristic of Down Syndrome. Immunoglobulin levels are present at reduced levels and T cell dysfunction has been shown in people with Down Syndrome.[2, 3, 4, 5, 6] The rate of infection in children with Down Syndrome is 52 times that of other children.[7] In fact, the immune system of a child with Down Syndrome is somewhat similar to the immune system of an adult over 65 years of age – lower numbers of overall white blood cells and a delayed immune system response.

In a study reported in the *Journal of the American Medical Association* (*JAMA*), the use of 200 units of vitamin E doubled the amount of white blood cell T lymphocytes and improved the immune system response to attack by seven times.[8]

Zinc, required by the thymus to produce white blood cells, and selenium which increases immunoglobulin, are low in children with Down Syndrome. Zinc prevents premature death of the white blood cells and lowers the number of infectious episodes in Down Syndrome.[9, 10, 11, 12, 13, 14, 15, 16, 17] Selenium has been shown to improve immunoglobulin levels in Down Syndrome. Zinc and selenium deficiencies are so well-documented in people with Down Syndrome that it is now recommended that these mineral levels be tested. However the laboratory measurement of zinc is not without problems: the common method is measuring plasma zinc which even the medical community acknowledges is not necessarily going to give an accurate assessment of zinc nutritional status.[18, 19, 20] Providing zinc supplements at doses at the RDA is proven safe and effective for people with Down Syndrome, and one study even showed that giving zinc can lower the number of infectious episodes, and result in improved school attendance.[21]

Studies demonstrate that in people with Down Syndrome, levels are also low of the antioxidant vitamins A, C and E, all of which are crucial for the immune system. Vitamin A has been shown to dramatically decrease the incidence of infection in Down Syndrome and is essential for maintenance of skin and mucous membranes. It also enhances white blood cell function and increases antibody response.

If we accept the argument that a weakened immune system is associated with aging, we can see what a weak immune system looks like by studying the elderly. And in fact this is where much of the research has been conducted. If we compare immune system damage in children with Down Syndrome, it mirrors that of an adult over 65 in terms of direct measurement of lymphocytes and antibody response.

We have lab studies in trisomic mice that show weakened immune systems, as well as demonstrated oxidative damage in children with Down Syndrome.[22, 23] Oxidative damage is the strongest evidence of immune system dysfunction because it indicates excessive free radicals. (For more on this, see Nutri-Chem's study in *Chapter 8*.)

While we see the evidence of weakened immune systems in Down Syndrome, and we know it's happening right from birth, the cause is still under investigation. But just as with other problems experienced by children with Down Syndrome, we don't need to prove the source in order to treat the symptoms. We don't withhold immune system therapy from the elderly while we study the phenomenon of aging. And we shouldn't do so in kids with Down Syndrome.

## Solutions: on your feet again

When you look back to the causes of immune system problems, you see that some are within our control: diet, sufficient rest, stress, smoking, excess radiation from the sun. So it's pretty obvious that you should eat well, get lots of sleep, don't smoke or stay out in the sun too long, alleviate stress (exercise is great for this) and so on. Other factors such as industrial pollution or pesticides in food may be beyond your control – all you can do is compensate for them as much as possible.

Nutrients play a dual role. They supply your immune system with essential ingredients to function, and they compensate for deficiencies created by external forces beyond your control. Your immune system has the most rapid turnover of cells in your body and is therefore most susceptible to nutritional deprivation. Contrast this with bone, where the cells are turning over slowly and the impact of bad nutrition takes longer to become apparent there.

Antioxidants provide a crucial defense against free radicals. While your body can produce enzymes to control free radicals and a good diet can contain antioxidant vitamins, it isn't enough when serious oxidative stress is present. Supplements are essential to nourish your immune system and to provide sufficient antioxidants to fight free radical damage.

Research involving elderly people showing signs of immune system dysfunction prove the power of antioxidants. In one study, vitamin E was administered to a group of elderly people. (It's noteworthy that vitamin E has only one role in our body – as an antioxidant – and is often called THE antioxidant vitamin.) The white blood cell count of the elderly people in the

# Vitamin A deficiency

Vitamin A has a proven role in immune system functioning and in reducing rates of infection in children with Down Syndrome. Vitamin A supplementation can reduce infant mortality among measles patients by at least 50% in third-world countries. However, in a study done among well-nourished children in California, they found that 50% of the children suffering from measles were deficient in vitamin A.

Prolonged vitamin A deficiency results in characteristic signs of folicular hypercarotosis. What this means is that there is a build up of cellular debris in the hair follicles giving the skin a goose bump appearance. Immune system abnormalities result in depressed antibody response, depressed levels of T cells and alteration in the gastrointestinal tract, lungs and respiratory tract.[24] This results in the gastro-intestinal tract, lungs and respiratory tract being more susceptible to infectious diseases. The deficiency of vitamin A may be because of inadequate intake or it may be as a result of some secondary factor that interferes with the absorption, storage or transport of vitamin A. Some of these factors that result in vitamin A deficiency include protein malnutrition and zinc deficiency. In fact, vitamin E and zinc are particularly important to the proper function of vitamin A. A deficiency of zinc, vitamin C, protein or thyroid hormone impairs the conversion of pro-vitamin A carotenes to vitamin A. Simple deficiency of carotenoids (the coloured compounds in fruits and vegetables that you get from your diet) is quite common. Consider that in one study, it was reported that 50% of children eat only one fruit or vegetable daily and that vegetable is french fries.

study rose, and their response to antigens increased by seven times.[25] If you think back to our army of defense, these seniors had more guns and they were seven times stronger so that they could pick up the artillery, aim it correctly and fire the trigger.

This study with seniors is but one of many proving the power of nutrition where our immune systems are concerned. The positive results were achieved with administration of only one antioxidant, vitamin E. Think what can happen when the whole army is deployed! A study conducted by Chandra, et al,[26, 27] in Newfoundland reported that the number of sick days in seniors were reduced by 50% using simple vitamin supplements. In Dr. Marie Peeters study of children with Down Syndrome using Nutri-Chem's MSB supplement, there was a reduction reported of 50% in the number of sick days.[28]

Nutrients are being studied in the general population for their benefits on the immune system for an important reason: antibiotics and other medical interventions don't work, and they carry serious risks and side effects. (In August, 2000, a *JAMA* study reported that 80,000 people died from infections introduced during hospital stays that could not be stopped by antibiotics.[29])

## The thyroid

The thyroid makes and stores thyroid hormones which regulate all of the body's processes including heart rate, blood pressure and the rate at which food is converted into energy (metabolism). Twenty-five percent of children with Down Syndrome have thyroid dysfunction (hypothyroidism). Insufficient thyroid hormone delays maturation of the bowel. If you can't burn energy – that is, use food – you don't grow. Hypothyroidism, especially during infancy and childhood, leads to depressed brain development, smaller stature, sluggishness and obesity. This gets compounded when weight becomes a problem, and children are placed on calorie-reduced diets that can further deplete the body's nutritional status.

Thyroid hormones also have an important role in intellectual development. It has been estimated that a newborn infant with untreated hypothyroidism will lose up to 5 I.Q. points each month during the first year of life.[30] But the broad range of symptoms associated with hypothyroidism make it difficult to diagnose in the very young, so parents may not know their child has a problem until damage has already been done. At Nutri-Chem, we recommend yearly monitoring for thyroid function by checking TSH, free T3 and free T4 levels with your doctor.

Hormones produced by the thyroid gland, located in the neck, regulate growth and metabolism in the body. Too much of these hormones (hyperthyroidism) or too little (hypothyroidism) can delay bowel development, alter heart rate and blood pressure, and affect mental state and brain development. Symptoms that point to a thyroid problem may include constipation, excess weight, low energy, decreased growth and development, or poor muscle tone. Disturbances in zinc and selenium can be fundamental to thyroid functioning.

Many of the same nutrients are involved in both thyroid function and immune system function. However, zinc is the only nutrient proven to improve thyroid function in Down Syndrome.[31, 32] It would then make sense that if zinc has been proven to regulate thyroid in Down Syndrome, you would use zinc before hormone therapy.

Additionally, vitamins E and A function together to manufacture active thyroid hormone. The active form of thyroid is actually T3 but it is made from T4 in the body and selenium is required to convert T4 to T3. Vitamin C and the B vitamins riboflavin (B2), niacin (B3) and pyridoxine (B6) are also necessary for normal thyroid hormone manufacture.

This chapter on the immune system and thyroid function demonstrate the intimate relationship between key nutrients deficient in Down Syndrome and the essential function of these systems. If a depressed thyroid function can suppress development of the brain and it has been shown that zinc and all the other mentioned nutrients can normalize thyroid function should it not be imperative that these nutrients are given importance and consideration in Down Syndrome?

## Closing comments from Kent:

*I recently spoke with a physician who told me that there is no evidence for vitamin therapy in Down Syndrome. I asked her if she had ever recommended zinc, vitamin A or a multi-vitamin for a child with Down Syndrome. No, she replied, never. What then, I asked her, do you give a child with Down Syndrome who has a recurring upper respiratory infection? Antibiotics, she said. This illustrates precisely how wrong-headed the approach to vitamins is with many doctors. They are antagonistic toward a safe vitamin supplement that has been proven effective such as zinc, yet readily prescribe drugs that weaken the immune system and do nothing for the infection.*

*Where is the sense in defending ineffective, unsafe drug therapies while refusing to offer safe and effective nutritional therapies? In my experience, such a position makes no sense. Common sense is found in the biochemical reality that there is no way to treat or stimulate the immune system other than through use of nutrients. – K.M.*

# Endnotes

1. http://www.cdc.gov/nip/vacsafe/concerns/thimerosal/faqs-mercury.htm

2. Anneren, G., et al. (1992) "Abnormal serum IgG subclass pattern in children with Down's syndrome." *Archives of Disease in Childhood* 67: 628-31.

3. Burgio, G.R., et al. (1975) "Derangements of immunoglobulin levels, phytohemagglutinin responsiveness and T and B cell markers in Down's syndrome at different ages." *European Journal of Immunology* 5: 600-603.

4. Bjorksten, B., et al. (1980) "Zinc and immune function in Down's syndrome." *Acta Paediatra Scand* 69: 183-187.

5. Fabris, N., et al. (1993) "Psychoendocrine – immune interactions in Down's Syndrome: Role of zinc. In: *Growth Hormone Treatment in Down's Syndrome* (ed. S. Castells and K.E. Wisniewski, John Wiley & Sons Ltd, London) p203-217.

6. Franceschi, C., et al. (1988) "Oral zinc supplementation in Down's syndrome: restoration of thymic endocrine activity and of some immune defects." *Journal of Mental Deficiency Research* 32: 169-181.

7. *Down Syndrome – Advances in Medical Care* (1992). Editors: Lott, I; McCoy, E.

8. Meydani, S., et al. (1997) "Vitamin E supplementation and in vivo immune response in healthy elderly subjects." *Journal of the American Medical Association* 277: 1380-86

9. Kadrabova, J., et al. (1996) "Changed serum trace element profile in Down's syndrome." *Biological Trace Element Research* 54: 201-206.

10. Lockitch, G., et al. (1989) "Infection and immunity in Down syndrome: A trial of long-term low oral doses of zinc." *Journal of Pediatrics* 114: 781-7.

11. Franceschi, C., et al. (1988) "Oral zinc supplementation in Down's syndrome: restoration of thymic endocrine activity and of some immune defects." *Journal of Mental Deficiency Research* 32: 169-181.

12. Bjorksten, B., et al. (1980) "Zinc and immune function in Down's syndrome." *Acta Paediatra Scand* 69: 183-187.

13. Anneren, G., et al. (1990) "Increase in serum concentrations of IgG2 and IgG4 by selenium supplementation in children with Down's syndrome." *Archives of Disease in Childhood* 65: 1353-1355.

14. Neve, J. et al. (1983) "Selenium, zinc and copper in Down's syndrome (trisomy 21): blood levels and relations with glutathione peroxidase and superoxide dismutase." *Clinica Chimica Acta* 133: 209-14.

15. Neve, J., et al. (1984) "Selenium and glutathione peroxidase in plasma and erythrocytes of Down's syndrome (trisomy 21) patients." *Journal of Mental Deficiency Research* 28: 261-68.

16. Griffiths, A., Behrman, J. (1967) "Dark adaptation in mongols." *Journal of Mental Deficiency Research* 11:23-30.

17. Shah, S., et al. (1989) "Antioxidant vitamin (A and E) status of down's syndrome subjects." *Nutrition Research* 9: 709-15.

18. Wood, J. (2000) "Assessment of Marginal Zinc Status in Humans." *Journal of Nutrition* 130:1350S-1354S.

19. Taylor, A. (1997) "Measurement of zinc in clinical samples." *Annals of Clinical Biochemistry* 34(Pt 2):142-50.

20. King, J.C. (1990) "Assessment of zinc status." *Journal of Nutrition* 120 Suppl 11:1474-9.

21. Fabris, N., et al. (1993) "Psychoendocrine – immune interactions in Down's syndrome: Role of zinc." In: *Growth Hormone Treatment in Down's syndrome* (ed. S. Castells and K.E. Wisniewski, John Wiley & Sons Ltd, London) p203-217.

22. Mirochnitchenko, Inouye M. (1996) "Effect of overexpression of human Cu,Zn superoxide dismutase in transgenic mice on macrophage functions." *Journal of Immunology* 1996 Feb 15;156(4):1578-86.

23. Jovanovic, S et al (1998) "Biomarkers of oxidative stress are significantly elevated in Down syndrome." *Free Radical Biology and Medicine* 25: 1044-48.

24. Palmer, S. (1978) "Influence of vitamin A nutriture on the immune response: findings in children with Down's syndrome." *International Journal of Vitamin and Nutrition Research* 48: 188-216

25. Meydani, S., et al. (1997) "Vitamin E supplementation and in vivo immune response in healthy elderly subjects." *Journal of the American Medical Association* 277: 1380-86

26. Chandra, R. (1992) "Effect of vitamin and trace-element supplementation on immune responses and infection in elderly subjects." *Lancet* 340: 1124-27.

27. Pike, J., and Chandra, R.K. (1995) "Effect of vitamin and trace element supplementation on immune indices in healthy elderly." *International Journal of Vitamin and Nutrition Research* 65: 117-20

28. Peeters, M., and MacLeod, K. (1999) Unpublished data. Reviewed in *Bridges* 4(1).

29. Starfield, B. (2000) "Is US Health Really the Best in the World?" *Journal of the American Medical Association* 284(4): 483-85.

30. Lindsay, R.S., and Toft, A.D. (1997) "Hypothyroidism." *Lancet* 349: 413-17.

31. Fabris, N., et al. (1993) "Psychoendocrine – immune interactions in Down's syndrome: Role of zinc." In: *Growth Hormone Treatment in Down's syndrome* (ed. S. Castells and K.E. Wisniewski, John Wiley & Sons Ltd, London) p203-217.

32. Franceschi, C., et al. (1988) "Oral zinc supplementation in Down's syndrome: restoration of thymic endocrine activity and of some immune defects." *Journal of Mental Deficiency Research* 32: 169-181.

# JACOB'S STORY

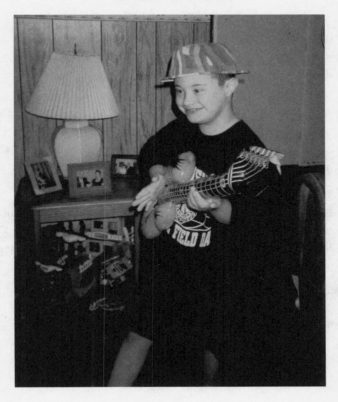

At six months of age, Jacob Spiegal developed infantile spasms. His mother Carol was asked to sign a release form acknowledging that she knew how dangerous the prescribed seizure medication could be for her baby – it could cause a brain aneurysm. When she looks back now more than six years later, she sees the irony of that situation.

"There they (doctors) were, pooh-poohing vitamins for children like Jacob with Down Syndrome. Yet I was being asked to sign a paper authorizing this horrible medicine that had all the side effects you could imagine," says Carol. "Jacob was cranky all the time on the drugs, gained a lot of weight, didn't sleep and had immune system problems."

While the medication did arrest most, but not all, of Jacob's seizures, Carol hoped for another solution. She found it when her son was nine months old.

"I saw a television show about vitamins for children with Down Syndrome and thought 'wow.' I started doing research because I'm one of those mums that, even though something looks good, I'm not prepared to put my child at risk." Jacob, now seven, has been taking MSB and piracetam ever since. In that time, Carol says, "he has not had one twitch of seizure."

Jacob has been so healthy, his mother says, that when he brought flu bugs home from school, his little sister Hannah, 5, got sick while Jacob remained well. "I phoned Nutri-Chem, and they sent a vitamin formula for Hannah," says Carol.

As a recent Grade One graduate, Jacob loves camping, swimming, dancing and music. "And he just adores his sister," says Carol. "And she him."

# CHAPTER 10

# THE BRAIN

*NO SUBJECT ASSOCIATED WITH DOWN SYNDROME RECEIVES MORE ATTENTION THAN THE BRAIN. Whether it's a question of IQ levels, mood disorders, dementia or early-onset Alzheimer's disease, the prognosis parents are given can be frightening. It's routine for parents to hear that their children will be mentally disabled and develop symptoms of Alzheimer's disease by their mid-thirties. These complex issues require explanation, but also perspective and an answer to the question: "Is there anything we can do?" And while I may be accused of skipping to the end of the mystery and revealing whodunit before you've read the details of the case, you'll be glad to know the answer is "yes!"*
*– K.M.*

## WHAT WILL I LEARN?

▸ How oxidation damages the brain.

▸ The link between Down Syndrome and Alzheimer's disease.

▸ What you can do to support optimum brain function.

# Getting inside your head

Your brain isn't just in charge of intelligence and emotions – it's also connected to bodily functions such as heartbeat and blood pressure and influences internal organs. Together with your spinal cord, it makes up what's called your central nervous system.

A roadmap of your brain would show three main areas (hindbrain, midbrain and forebrain), each with its own role in specific functions of your body. Sensory nerve cells feed information from every part of your body to your brain which processes this data and sends out instructions through nerve cells. This complex communications system functions like central command over an army that is comprised of your body's physical, emotional and intellectual foot soldiers. It can order the squadron in charge of walking to start or stop, the emotional platoon to laugh or cry and the intellectual battalion to solve a mathematical problem or store information in the memory bank for later.

Brain cells are special – more complex than other cells in our body, but also more susceptible to oxidation, a chemical reaction that damages and destroys these very cells. Because of this, our brains can age and deteriorate before our bodies do. Sometimes

## DEFINING MOMENT

**Fatty acids:** organic acids found in fats and oils

**Saturated fats:** solid fats that have all their carbon atoms saturated with hydrogen

**Unsaturated fats:** liquid fats with empty spaces because of missing hydrogen atoms

**Polyunsaturated fats:** fats saturated with two or more hydrogen atoms

**Hydrogen:** key component of many biological/organic molecules in our bodies; can also be a very powerful free radical

**Oxygen:** required for breathing; essential element that is a key component of many biological/organic molecules in our bodies; extremely chemically active

**Oxidation:** when an atom or molecule loses electrons, it is oxidized; (i.e. when an antioxidant steals an electron from a fat, the fat has been oxidized)

**Hydrogenation:** process of oxidation that turns liquid fat into solid fat by saturating it (heating) with hydrogen

**Down Syndrome and Vitamin Therapy**

known as premature aging, the real term for this programmed cell death is apoptosis.

## Essential elements and essential fatty acids:

We live in a "fat phobic" world where grocery stores contain an endless array of foods trumpeted as "lowfat" or "nonfat". In this environment, it seems contradictory to recommend supplements of essential fatty acids (EFAs). But here's why you should.

You need essential elements – oxygen, hydrogen, carbon, nitrogen and sulfur – in large quantities. The good news is that you get them in large quantities in the food you eat and the very air you breathe. This is not the case for Essential Fatty Acids (EFA). It sounds counter-intuitive: it seems that fats are everywhere in our modern diet, and our bodies can convert proteins and carbohydrates into fats if needed. EFAs, however, are fats needed by the membranes that surround the cells in your body. While other fats are easily obtained from food, food – with the exception of certain oils, seeds and nuts – is a poor source of EFAs. Although we should consume no more than 30% of our daily calories as fats, a lack of essential fatty acids presents a serious health threat. (Experts estimate that approximately 80% of our population consumes insufficient EFAs.) While EFAs have many roles in maintaining healthy skin, blood pressure, cholesterol levels and blood clotting, one of the most important functions of EFAs is in the brain.

## The skinny on fat

Your brain is comprised mainly of fat (estimates range as high as 60%), found in the cell membranes which surround the cell nucleus where genes and chromosomes reside. Brain cells are unsaturated liquid fats (lipids), highly organized with all the molecules lined up like a group of magnets all facing the same direction. The organic acids found in fats (called fatty acids) have a role in the brain's structure, and also how it functions. They are the traffic cops dictating the movement of neurotransmitters (chemicals such as acetycholine, dopamine and serotonin that transmit nerve impulses between cells).

Essential fatty acids (EFAs), omega-3 and omega-6, are known as parent lipids whose offspring make up half of your brain lipids. Approximately one-quarter of these are in the form of DHA (docosahexaenoic acid), an essential ingredient in breast milk and also present in the membranes of the retina. (You may have heard about recent studies supporting the addition of essential fatty acids and DHA in infant formulas, something that several countries outside North America have now done.)

Research into the omega-3 fatty acid EPA (eicosapentaenoic acid) has shown it has an important role in the functioning of the brain. Controlled studies out of Harvard have shown that EPA supplementation has dramatic benefits for depression.[1] While we cannot take samples of the brain while someone is alive, it has been shown that the red blood cell membrane mirrors the structure of the membranes of the brain. Studies have shown alterations and deficiencies in red blood cell fatty acids of individuals with Alzheimer's disease. We have observed in our Nutri-Chem lab work, almost universally depressed levels of omega-3 fatty acids in red blood cells of kids with Down Syndrome. However, we do not know if this is as a result of dietary deficiency or genetics.[2, 3] Other cofactors such as zinc, magnesium, B6, vitamin C and niacin are essential for the correct biotransformation of essential fatty acids. So again we have an example of how all nutrients work together in that deficiencies in these cofactors will cause disturbances in essential fatty acids.

In addition to the connection to mental disease, there are over 60 health conditions that can benefit from essential fatty acid supplementation. For this reason I recommend red blood cell membrane testing for composition of fatty acids.

## From the fat into the fire

One of the most common places you encounter the results of a process called hydrogenation is in your supermarket. Here, the shelves are full of food products that have been made with hydrogenated oils. One of these is margarine, created through a process of heating oil that turns it solid. The result is saturated fat – the very same artery-clogging substance your doctor has warned you about.

Sophisticated chefs say that if you understand chemistry, you understand cooking. Actions and reactions of chemical elements dictate whether a cake rises tall in the oven, or falls flat. In our bodies, the same chemistry (called biochemistry) is at work. Electrons from free radicals (highly chemically-reactive atoms that cause cell damage) blast the sensitive, organized unsaturated brain fats, rendering them disorganized and useless. Oxidation creates extra unattached molecules which act like wrecking balls destroying anything in their path as they keep on going.

In your kitchen, an overcooked cake isn't a tragedy (although if it's a six-year-old's birthday cake, they might disagree). In your brain, however, oxidation will disturb and destroy the healthy fats, in particular the omega fatty acids necessary for structure and function.

## Cleaning up the mess

If you've ever had a souffle explode in your oven, you know that it leaves you with a pretty big cleanup job. The same thing happens in your body when hydrogen from free radicals reacts with chemicals such as oxygen and oxidation results. This is not a tidy or easily-controlled process. There will be sparks flying –

the more oxidation, the more sparks are created. Fortunately, nature has given us some powerful protection against the fire of oxidation and the clean-up rags we need for the debris left behind. These are the antioxidants that work by grabbing free radicals (sparks) and neutralizing them before they can do more damage, then mopping up the mess.

Another way of understanding this process is to think of a small grease fire that is difficult to put out and superoxide dismutase (SOD) turns (or dismutes) this hard-to-put-out grease fire into a series of small fires that are easier to put out. However, the body can't cope with the extra number of small fires that are being created by this extra chromosome. Down Syndrome individuals have more fires and yet they have the same number of firefighters as the non-Down Syndrome population – their bodies can't cope with this number of fires. This results in a constant imbalance in their oxidative chemistry.

Vitamin E, an antioxidant, is most reactive against hydroxyl free radicals. It absorbs them, sacrificing itself in the process. Ginkgo biloba, an antioxidant herb, improves glutathione, a protein that acts like a wash rag inside the cell. Selenium works with vitamin E and washes the dirty glutathione rag so it can be recycled and used again. SOD is one of the enzymes that acts as a cleanup rag, grabbing the massive amounts of superoxide free radicals generated through oxidation. This happens at an intermediate stage of a cycle where peroxyl radicals are formed and catalase, another antioxidant enzyme, turns these into harmless water.

## Oxidation and Down Syndrome

In Down Syndrome, there is more SOD (called overexpression) because the gene for SOD is found on the 21st chromosome. Oxidative stress may result from this excess SOD because in the process of it controlling the superoxide radical, hydrogen peroxide is generated creating hydroxyl free radicals. SOD is also implicated in increasing peroxyl radicals at the point where catalase is converting these peroxyl radicals into water. It's like this extra copy of a gene (the one spinning out SOD) is a tiger in the woods with his tail on fire, lighting fires as he goes. Now there's more fire, but still the same amount of water in the bucket to put out the fires.

The effect of this ongoing oxidation isn't lethal but it creates constant destruction. As oxidation occurs, it saturates and destabilizes fats in brain cells. This increased amount of oxidative stress (or the imbalance of fires) is implicated in Alzheimer's disease, cataracts, cancer, heart disease, autoimmune diseases and virtually any disease of a chronic, debilitating nature.

## The Alzheimer's link

Alzheimer's disease is the culmination of a degenerative process that happens in the brain. Nerve cells where thought processes take place degenerate and die. In addition, chemicals in the brain that carry messages to and from the nerve cells (neurotransmitters) are lowered, resulting in disruptions to thinking and memory.

Before someone is diagnosed as having Alzheimer's disease, they may have behaviour or mood disorders, deteriorating mental functions or dementia. These are really symptoms, not diseases in themselves.

To make a diagnosis of Alzheimer's disease, neuropsychological testing is used that measures function in a number of areas, including personality and mood changes. However, the brain structure characteristic of Alzheimer's can't be measured until an autopsy is performed – in other words, after a person has died. It is only when we look at the brain that we can see the plaques and tangles considered the markers of the disease.

# Will your child develop Alzheimer's?

Parents are commonly told that by the age of 35 to 40, all people with Down Syndrome exhibit the plaques and tangles in their brains that signify Alzheimer's disease. Does this mean that all people with Down Syndrome eventually get Alzheimer's?

Dementia has several causes. Alzheimer's is one, but vascular disease (causing strokes), Lewy bodies (structures from proteins that develop inside nerve cells causing their degeneration), Pick's Disease (brain cell degeneration localized in frontal lobe), infection (Creutzfeldt-Jakob Disease or Mad Cow Disease), toxins (including those from chemicals found in environmental pollutants or prescription drugs) and head injuries all cause symptoms of dementia. In addition, dementia-like symptoms can result from depression and other mental health problems.

Researchers studying Alzheimer's in people with Down Syndrome are now questioning whether the neurological characteristics symptomatic of Alzheimer's (brain plaques and tangles) do in fact lead inevitably to progressive dementia caused by this disease. Studies have reported findings indicating that the incidence of progressive dementia and Alzheimer's is much lower than previously thought in Down Syndrome[4, 5, 6]. In addition, depression can account for a decline in mental functioning and changes in behaviour.

Aging experts postulate that if we live long enough, we all get Alzheimer's because our brain cells die of natural causes. As our immune system wears out, free radicals attack our brains cells which are high in fat content and particularly vulnerable to hydrogenation (oxidation).

Whether or not it's true that all people with Down Syndrome get Alzheimer's disease, it's undeniable that degeneration is happening causing serious changes in the brain, and it's happening right from birth. If symptoms of dementia are present – loss of self-care, lower verbal and social skills, withdrawal, aggressive behaviour, changes in sleep patterns, forgetfulness –

the quality of life for a person with Down Syndrome will be diminished. And it will happen at an earlier age than in the general population.

## The genetic link

One way to attempt to understand the genetic link between Alzheimer's and Down Syndrome is to look at the genetic link between Alzheimer's disease and the non-Down Syndrome population. A landmark study done after the second world war followed 500 pairs of identical twins and concluded that Alzheimer's disease was NOT genetically determined.[7] The study reported that a significant number of the identical twin sets had one who developed Alzheimer's and one who did not. The study concluded that Alzheimer's disease was an environmental disorder with a genetic susceptibility. Since then, researchers have been searching for the environmental link to Alzheimer's.

## Is oxidative stress the culprit?

The most compelling environmental causes that are of interest to those of us concerned with Down Syndrome revolve around oxidative stress. Perry et al [8, 9] showed increased levels of oxidative stress in the brains of Down Syndrome individuals with Alzheimer's disease. In the study in *Nature* [10] on oxidative stress, vitamin E was shown in vitro to prevent premature cell death of brain cells. When you added vitamin E to the brain cells of Down Syndrome individuals, the brain cells grew and thrived (see *Chapter 4* for more on this study).

In the first ever in vivo study, the International Center for Metabolic testing Laboratory (ICMT) looked at approximately 166 Down syndrome individuals and their siblings as controls.[11] Blood and urine analysis showed increased levels of oxidative stress in individuals with Down Syndrome, and low levels of antioxidants and low levels of glutathione.

# Antioxidants to the rescue

The use of antioxidants in people with Down Syndrome to prevent Alzheimer's disease makes sense, yet it has not been studied. It is noteworthy that the American Psychiatric Society has recommended only three substances as standard of care in Alzheimer's based on controlled studies. Two of these substances are antioxidants – vitamin E and Ginkgo Biloba – and the third substance is the Aricept class of drugs.

In addition to the work of Perry et al, the evidence which shows increased levels of oxidative stress in the brains of individuals with Down Syndrome and Alzheimer's disease is simply the fact that vitamin E[12] will improve the course of Alzheimer's disease. Vitamin E has no biological role other than as an antioxidant.

Ginkgo Biloba has also been proven to delay the progression of Alzheimer's.[13] Ginkgo Biloba has direct antioxidant properties and has been shown to increase levels of glutathione (see section later in this chapter).

We know there is oxidative stress in Alzheimer's disease and in Down Syndrome. We also know that antioxidants have been shown to alter the course of Alzheimer's. Despite this, however, the criticism of vitamin E and Gingko Biloba for use in Alzheimer's is that the effects are significant but not dramatic. This suggests that there is a toxic element in the brain. In other words, how can you give all these antioxidants and not see a reversal of the situation (Alzheimer's) and not just a slowed progression of the disease. This leads us to examine another factor that has an impact on oxidative stress – heavy metals.

# The mercury connection

Heavy metals can cause damage in the brain such as Alzheimer's disease. They can cause oxidative damage, reduce glutathione and lower levels of antioxidants.

One of the most compelling toxins to examine in the brain is the heavy metal mercury. The effects of mercury occur on the most abundant protein in the brain which is called tubulin.

Mercury interferes with the sulfhydryl groups in tubulin of which there are at least 13 sites per protein molecule. Blocking of these sites by mercury has been shown to destroy the brain cell and cause its collapse.[14, 15, 16] This effect can be caused by only one molecule of mercury. Its effect is like pulling out the bottom can from a stacked up pile of cans, causing the entire structure to collapse. Likewise this one molecule of mercury can destroy a complete structure of a brain cell. Think of the effects over a lifetime.

## The glutathione defense

Luckily the body has protection in the guise of scavenging sulphydryl peptides and proteins. In other words we have have this defense network that excretes heavy metals from our system. One of the crucial sulphydryl scavengers is glutathione – the main intracellular antioxidant. If glutathione levels are low, the brain is more susceptible to attack by these heavy metal toxins.

Glutathione has many roles. One is that of an intracellular antioxidant that is recycled and reactivated by extracellular (outside the cell) antioxidants such as vitamin C, vitamin E, coenzyme Q10, carotenoids and other food-based antioxidants found in fruits and vegetables.

Glutathione also acts as a protector against toxins by sacrificing itself to remove heavy metals. The enzymatic reactivation of glutathione via selenium in the form of selenocystein is part of glutathione peroxidase (an enzyme which recycles and reactivates gluthathione). You need adequate levels of the antioxidant selenium for the enzymatic reactivation of glutathione. As explained in *Chapter 7*, selenium has been shown to improve the immune system in Down Syndrome which is highly sensitive to oxidative stress and heavy metal toxicity. In this, we see a logical connection to how all these elements work together.

Glutathione is such a good antioxidant because it so easily receives and donates an electron. It's like a sponge that quickly soaks up water or debris which is easily gotten rid of when you squeeze the sponge. This function is useful in many processes besides that of an antioxidant. It is used in the most basic metabolism, thus helping to eliminate toxins including heavy metals. (Heavy metals and the drug tylenol depress glutathione because glutathione is used up instead detoxifying and removing the heavy metals and drugs.)

Glutathione is worthy of specific note because it has a pivotal role in so many processes in the body relevant to Down Syndrome. These are:

- as an antioxidant;
- its use in the energy cycle (Kreb's cycle);
- acting as a sponge to recycle and clean itself;
- phase 2 elimination, which is how the body excretes heavy metals and other toxins.

## Glutathione and Down Syndrome

Children with Down Syndrome have low levels of glutathione. The solution seems simple: just give more glutatione as a supplement. If only it were that simple! The problem is that your body doesn't absorb glutathione very well. Even if glutathione is in your blood, it has to somehow get past intrastitial fluid inside the cell. To just give more glutathione would be like spraying water on the outside of your house to water your plants inside the house.

So how do you improve the levels of glutathione? One of the simplest ways is also the most effective. Take vitamin C. Vitamin C will recycle glutathione. Vitamin C will work synergistically with vitamin E, coenzyme Q10, selenium and other antioxidants such as carotenoids, zinc, manganese, vitamin A and the amino acids cysteine, taurine and glycine.

Let's return to the landmark study where 500 pairs of identical twins were followed and one twin developed Alzheimer's disease and the other didn't. We don't know if the one twin developed the disease because they didn't have adequate antioxidants or because their brain was exposed to an environmental toxin like mercury. Or was it simply a subtle combination of inadequate antioxidants and environmental toxins?

It is remarkable that it has been argued that mercury exposure should only be limited in individuals whose biochemical make-up suggests a susceptibility. This is tantamount to arguing that only a child with asthma should not be exposed to tobacco smoke. The onus should be put directly on the offender to remove proven and noxious substances for everyone. If it is poisonous, then it should be removed.

## What's to be done?

Research is increasing into the causes of dementia including Alzheimer's disease, most notably with regard to our rapidly-aging population. While this research is important, we have safe, non-drug tools now to fight oxidation and the symptoms of dementia it causes. These are found in antioxidants, in particular vitamin E, DHA, Gingko Biloba, and the essential fatty acids (EFAs) needed for optimum brain function. We also need to test for other possible causes of mental deterioration and mood disorders: anemia, thyroid problems and side effects from medications.

# Closing comments from Kent:

*Vitamin E is considered a protection against Alzheimer's disease, not a prevention. Doctors routinely say that "vitamin E is not a cure" for Alzheimer's disease, but what they're looking at is short-term usage long after the problem of oxidation has begun. If you want to prevent a car from rusting, you have to use a little oil regularly and you have to start before the problem happens. It's the same with antioxidants.*

*You can have short-term improvements with antioxidants in the immune and digestive systems – not in the brain. You have to start early because once brain deterioration happens, it's too late to reverse it. If we want to determine whether or not antioxidants can be preventive, not just protective, when it comes to brain deterioration, we'll need long-term studies conducted for periods of 20 to 30 years. In the meantime, protection is reason enough to justify using antioxidants as early in life as possible.*

*It is important to have perspective when looking at a degenerative neurological disease like Alzheimer's. While it is one of the most costly and devastating diseases facing society, we have hardly any studies on any substances that have a dramatic impact on this disease.*

*The studies that do exist have shown that antioxidants such as vitamin E, Ginkgo Biloba and the class of aricept-like drugs are of benefit. No controlled studies have been done on any substance with respect to preventing cognitive decline or Alzheimer's disease in Down Syndrome.*

*With this in mind, I have provided a table of nutrients and drugs outlining their benefits in Alzheimer's disease, their limitations, their function, risks and adverse effects, established long-term safety and whether they are biologically complementary. – K.M.*

# Therapeutic Choices in Dementia and Alzheimer's Disease

## 1. Goals of Therapy:

- to slow disease progression
- to treat behavioural problems
- to treat concomitant depression
- to alleviate caregiver burden

## 2. Listed pharmacologic choices:

**TACRINE** – A cholinesterase inhibitor, with hepatic toxicity. Only approved in the U.S.A.

**ARICEPT** – A cholinesterase inhibitor with a higher specificity for centrally active cholinesterase than tacrine. Side effects are cholinergic in nature, e.g., nausea, vomiting and diarrhea. Hepatic toxicity has not been reported. Dose range: 5 to 10 mg. A 12-week trial has shown benefits with patients having mild to moderate Alzheimer's disease. (*Dementia* 1996; 7:293-303)

**VITAMIN E** – A dose of 2000 IU per day of the alpha-tocopherol form has demonstrated evidence for benefit in disease progression. A few side effects were apparent beyond an increased incidence of falls. (*N Engl J Med* 1997; 336:1216-1222) Vitamin E also serves to protect dietary essential fatty acids (EFA).

**ANTIDEPRESSANTS** – Many patients in the early stages suffer from depression. More "activating" antidepressants (SSRI) are recommended, because they are less likely to cause anticholinergic side effects or to worsen orthostatic hypotension.

**TRAZODONE** – as a serotonergic agonist, is often used to manage agitated behaviour (*Psychopharmacology*. New York: Raven, 1995: 1427-1436)

**BENZODIAZEPINES** – Data on their efficacy is conflicting. They can reduce agitation, but can also lead into over-sedation and worsening cognition.

**NEUROLEPTICS** – Have been replaced by non-neuroleptics as first-line treatment. Good studies are lacking, although they have been used for many years. As the elderly brain is exquisitely sensitive to neuroleptics, Initial doses should be small. "Start low, go slow" Neuroleptic induced akathisia (increased motor restlessness) may be interpreted as lack of drug effect. The dose then is increased, increasing motor restlessness. A vicious cycle leading to extrapyramidal rigidity to the point of immobility.

**MISC.** – Beta-blockers (particularly pindolol), carbamazepine, lithium and buspirone have also been used in case reports, but evidence is lacking.

### 3. Additional nutritional choices:

**ASA** – Acetylsalicylic acid has been reported to slow progression of multi-infarct dementia.

**EFA'S** – Manipulation of dietary fats, by using essential fatty acids, is a proven therapy to reduce formation of arachidonic acid and thus inflammation. Vitamin E works synergistically. (*Med. Hypothesis* 50: 335-37, 1998)

**GINKGO BILOBA** – Increases oxygen uptake and blood flow in the capillary system of cerebral and peripheral circulation. In addition, perhaps most importantly, it has antioxidant potential, reducing the damaging activity of free radicals. This study also emphasized that Ginkgo enhances cognition and improves daily living and social behaviour. (A placebo-controlled, double-blind randomized trial on Ginkgo extract in Dementia, *JAMA*, 278(16):1327-32,1997)

**GLUTATHIONE** – Glutathione serves as one of the primary brain antioxidants. So that its deficiency would potentially allow increased free radical damage. (*Biochemical Pharmacology* 25:52 (8): 1147-54, 1996)

**LIPOIC ACID** – Lipoic acid is a powerful antioxidant that is rapidly absorbed from the gut and readily enters the brain to protect neurons from free radical damage. Furthermore, it recycles the Vitamins C, E and glutathione. (*Iron and Oxidative Damage in Neurodegenerative Disease*, Beal, M.F. (ed.), New York, Wiley-Liss Pub. 1997)

**NAC** – N-Acetyl-Cysteine, orally applied, enhances the production of glutathione. In addition, it plays an antioxidant role itself. It especially reduces one of the most notorious free radicals in Alzheimer's disease, nitric oxide, by reducing the activity of nitric oxide synthetase. (*Free Radical biology and Medicine* 24(1): 39-48, 1997)

**COQ10** – Coenzyme Q10 is a critical transporter of electrons in the process of energy production of every living cell. I could enhance energy production in brain neurons. (Lass, Sohal, *Free Radical Biology*, 27(1/2):220-26,1999)

**ACETYL-L-** – It functions primarily as a shuttle, transporting fatty acids

**CARNITINE** – as "fuel" into the mitochondria. A second task is to facilitate the removal of toxic byproducts of brain metabolism. It can be converted into the neurotransmitter, acetylcholine, which is known to be profoundly deficient in the brains of Alzheimer's patients. A study at the University of California showed a striking reduction in the rate of mental decline in younger Alzheimer's patients, taking acetyl-l-carnitine over 1 year. (*Neurology* 47:705-711, 1996)

**PHOSPHATIDYL- SERINE** – Over the past two decades extensive medical literature has appeared, describing the important role of lecithin for brain function. More recent research revealed, that the beneficial action is due to only one component in lecithin, phosphatidylserine! It is one of the essential constituents of neuronal membranes, but it also a basic requirement to maintain vital energy production of the mitochondria. (*Neurology* 41:644 – 49, 1991)

**SAM-CYCLE** – In a study, published in the *Lancet*, May 8,1999, from the Department of Neurology and Clinical Chemistry at the University of Heidelberg, researchers revealed, that the second most frequent cause of dementia in the elderly population was "vascular dementia," caused by homocysteine elevation. Homocysteine is metabolized in the Sam-Cycle, using B6, B12, betain and folic acid as cofactors. The conclusion of this report provided very strong support for the effectiveness of B-complex and folic acid supplementation in terms of reducing risk of dementia. (*Lancet* 3531 586 – 87, 1999)

**PENTOXIFYLLINE** – OTC drug in Germany for decades, decreases blood viscosity, improves fluidity of erythrocytes, improves microcirculation and inhibits thrombocyte-aggregation. (*Mutschler, Pharmacology*, 1996)

**PIRACETAM** – A nootropic agent. Its mechanism of action is so far poorly defined. Some investigators use the term "metabolic enhancer", others suggest, that it "selectively improves the efficiency of higher telencephalic integrative activities." (Tacconi & Wurtmann, 1986; Klawans & Genovese, 1986) Nicholson, 1990; suggest that its primary action is to improve learning and memory. Piracetam is a cyclic gamma-aminobutyric acid (GABA) derivative, with no GABA-ergic effects. Under both normal and hypoxic conditions, piracetam has been reported to increase levels of adenosine triphosphate (ATP) in the brain, which has been suggested as the potential mechanism of action to explain some of the beneficial effects. (Branconnier, 1983; Nicholson, 1990) Controlled studies to date have not provided convincing evidence that piracetam alone or in combination with lecithin or choline is consistently effective in improving cognition or memory function in Alzheimer-type dementia. (*Growdon et al.* 1986)

# Endnotes

1. Andrew Stoll (2000) *The Omega-3 Connection: How you can Restore your Body's Natural Balance and Treat Depression.* Simon & Schuster

2. Brooksbank, B.W.L., and Martinez, M. (1989) "Lipid Abnormalities in the brain in adult Down's syndrome and Alzheimer's Disease." In: *Molecular and Chemical Neuropathology* Ed. L.A. Horrocks, The Humana Press Inc.

3. Pastor, M.C., et al. "Antioxidant enzymes and fatty acid status in erythrocytes of Down's syndrome patients" (1998) *Clinical Chemistry* 44(5): 924-929

4. Wisniewski, H.M., and Rabe, A. (1985) "Discrepancy between Alzheimer-type neuropathology and dementia in persons with Down syndrome." *Annals of the New York Academy of Sciences* 477: 247-260.

5. Janicki, M.P., and Dalton, A.J. (2000). "Prevalence of dementia and impact on intellectual disability services." *Mental Retardation* 38: 277-289.

6. Janicki, M.P., et al. (1996) "Practice guidelines for the clinical assessment and care management of Alzheimer's disease and other dementias among adults with intellectual disability." *Journal of Intellectual Disability Research* 40: 374-382.

7. Breitner J.C., et al. (1995) "Alzheimer's disease in the National Academy of Sciences-National Research Council Registry of Aging Twin Veterans. III. Detection of cases, longitudinal results, and observations on twin concordance." *Archives of Neurology.* 52(8):763-71

8.. Odetti, P., et al. (2000) "Early glycoxidation damage in brains from Down's syndrome." *Biochemical and Biophysical Research Communications* 243: 849; 1998.

9. Nunomura A., et al. (2000) "Neuronal oxidative stress precedes amyloid-ß deposition in Down syndrome." *Journal of Neuropathology and Experimental Neurology* 59, 1011-1017.

10. Busciglio, J., and Yanker, B. (1995) "Apoptosis and increased generation of reactive oxygen species in Down's syndrome neurons in vitro." *Nature* 378: 776-779.

11. Jovanovic, S., et al. (1998) "Biomarkers of oxidative stress are significantly elevated in Down syndrome." *Free Radical Biology and Medicine* 25: 1044-48.

12. Sano, M., et al. (1997) "A controlled trial of selegiline, alpha-tocopherol, or both as treatment for Alzheimer's disease." *New England Journal of Medicine* 336: 1216-22.

13. Le Bars P.L., et al. (1997) "A placebo-controlled, double-blind, randomized trial of an extract of Ginkgo Biloba for dementia. North American EGb Study Group." *Journal of the American Medical Association.* 278(16):1327-32.

14. Pendergrass J.C., et al. (1997) "Mercury vapor inhalation inhibits binding of GTP to tubulin in rat brain: similarity to a molecular lesion in Alzheimer diseased brain." *Neurotoxicology.* 18(2):315-24.

15. Palkiewicz P., et al. (1194) "ADP-ribosylation of brain neuronal proteins is altered by in vitro and in vivo exposure to inorganic mercury." *Journal of Neurochemistry.* 62(5):2049-52.

16. Vogel D.G., et al. (1985) "The effects of methyl mercury binding to microtubules." *Toxicology and Applied Pharmacology.* 80(3):473-86.

# SECTION 4

# WHAT PARENTS NEED TO KNOW ABOUT TESTS

## CHAPTER 11
### A Parent's Guide to Reading Studies and Blood Tests

## CHAPTER 12
### One mother's story

# WILLIAM'S STORY

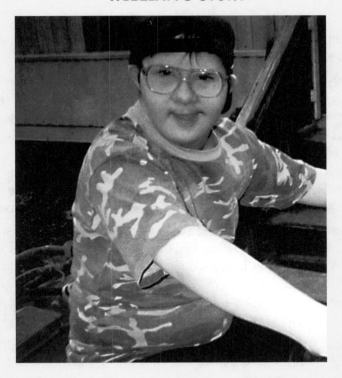

For William Musselwhite's mother Donna, every day is "a surprise, an adventure and a blessing." That's because 13-year-old William is always coming up with some new talent or accomplishment that delights his parents and large extended family – working on his new computer, singing gospel music in a choir or helping his father Bill with his woodcrafts. All of this defies the predictions of his early doctors.

"William was born two months prematurely," says Donna. "We didn't know he had Down Syndrome until he was three weeks old. The doctor told us to put him in an institution because William would never be capable of doing anything." Three months later when Donna complained about her baby's breathing, she was told it was nothing – she was simply a "neurotic mother." The truth emerged after William stopped breathing and it was discovered he had a hole in his heart and his lungs were filling with blood.

Surgery took care of William's heart problem, but he continued to experience constant sickness for the first several years of his life. "If someone sneezed around him, William got sick," his mother recalls. When her son was five, Donna heard about nutritional supplements and decided to investigate. She was already convinced about his potential to learn based on how alert and interested in his environment he had become. She contacted Nutri-Chem and asked a lot of questions. He started on MSB a few months later.

"When William started on the supplements, he could say only a few words like 'mama, daddy, go, bye bye.' Not long after, Bill was down on the floor looking for something he'd lost when William said, 'Daddy, what are you doing?'. Bill just froze and called me since William had never used a sentence before. Since then William has been talking in sentences."

With the help of William's older sister, Donna has home-schooled her son after the local school said they couldn't accommodate him in a regular classroom. He is active socially in his church and community, and has a special friendship with the 15-year-old daughter of his mother's friend. Donna says that the contrast between William and his friend Leatha (who does not take vitamin supplements) is dramatic. "William is almost never sick while Leatha has a lot of health problems including thyroid and breathing difficulties."

William likes to read and he loves music, friends and his dog, Donna says. His self-esteem is high and he's outspoken with his opinions. "William has taught us so much. He's so special, and so loving. We feel that we're blessed."

# CHAPTER 11

# A PARENT'S GUIDE TO READING STUDIES AND BLOOD TESTS

*AS SCIENTISTS WE SEEK TRUTH and conducting studies is part of how we find it. That said, however, the more I am involved with existing studies the more I see that they consist of "lies, damn lies and statistics." Therein lies the problem.*

*The purpose of a study is to prove or disprove something, and that is how researchers approach studies from the outset. In other words, the very intent predetermines the outcome (i.e. that the thing being studied is of value or is of no value).*

*Where vitamin studies are concerned, the number of people who want to study their effectiveness is a function of the environment we find ourselves in at this time. For example, 20 years ago medicine and doctors believed that we would find an antibiotic to kill every infection and research focused on finding these drug cures. Today, however, the public is actually examining the behaviour of physicians as to why we are giving antibiotics for infections for which they have no effect (bronchitis, upper respiratory infections, colds and so-called ear infections). We now have public campaigns saying "stop overusing antibiotics!"*

**WHAT WILL I LEARN?**

▸ How to decipher medical studies and blood tests.

▸ The single most important fact you need to know when reading a medical study.

▸ Advice from parents on how to get the information you need from your child's doctor.

From this evolution we see a transition in the bias of 20 years ago that favoured drugs as against nutritional therapies. So we see that bias is also a function of timing. Today researchers are looking to safe biological interventions such as vitamins as an effective alternative to drug therapies.

If we look at nutrients in this context of bias and the biological approach to the immune system in Down Syndrome, we need look no further than simple vitamin A. In the 1970s, Palmer et al[1] reported a dramatic decrease in infection rates in Down Syndrome with the use of vitamin A. This is an example of a significant study showing good reduction in infection rates using safe levels of a specific vitamin. Sounds simple, correct? Wrong! There was no economic incentive to promote and study vitamin A and this simple, safe and inexpensive concept of using vitamin A to reduce infections was not promoted or studied further.

The medical response to the Palmer study was to investigate vitamin A absorption in Down Syndrome. If they could prove that vitamin A absorption is not altered in Down Syndrome, then they could prove that vitamin A is not a problem in Down Syndrome. How does this relate to the issue of vitamin A and infections?! Yet the focus on studying absorption effectively shut down any further discussion of vitamin A's efficacy in fighting infections.

**Vaccinations:** Another illustration of research bias and biological interventions can be found in the case of vaccinations. In Ontario, Canada, there is a program to provide free flu vaccines to all residents. There are significant numbers of adverse reactions to flu vaccines with extremely questionable evidence of their benefit.

The evidence from two studies indicates that there is an approximately 50% chance of predicting in advance which flu bug is going to infect a population. Yet we have a massive vaccination program. Thimerosal (which is 50% ethyl mercury) is the preservative in these vaccinations. (See Chapter 9 for more on this.) Basically what we have done with this response is to introduce toxic metals and adverse reactions into the population with no better than chance odds of preventing flu.

Contrast this with evidence from full double blind placebo controlled trials demonstrating a 50% reduction of sick days in the senior population, as well as a seven-fold improvement in the immune response of seniors, with vitamin E alone and no adverse effects.[2]

The World Health Organization has shown a significant reduction in mortality from measles with the use of vitamin A in third-world countries.[3] This same benefit has been shown in the U.S. as well in Northern California.[4] Meanwhile all our resources seem to be directed toward vaccinating children against measles. This is occurring where current rates of adverse reactions reported to the VAERS (Vaccine Adverse Event Reporting System) exceed the number of infections caused by the vaccines used to prevent the viruses.

The vitamin A and nutrient connection is ignored despite U.S. Department of Agriculture reports of widespread vitamin A deficiency.[5] What we see is that a safe, simple and inexpensive nutrient is ignored in favour of a multi-billion dollar vaccination and drug industry.

I recently sat on a panel discussing the safety of vaccinations in Ontario. It was interesting to note that during the discussions there was no disagreement from any professional on the panel including government health officials about the adverse reactions and the doubt of efficacy of these vaccinations. As a matter of fact we were all in agreement including the government health officials on many of the issues I have raised in the above paragraphs. Furthermore, the government health officers acknowledged that the widespread use of a flu vaccine in Ontario was politically motivated and not health motivated. What this in effect does is raise the issue of credibility. The government of the day thought the public would perceive that the state was concerned about the health of the public by physically administering a free vaccine for which it ultimately has the support and financial incentives for physicians, pharmacists, nurses and the pharmaceutical industry. It makes everyone look good!

In addition to all of this we see one of the most disturbing editorials ever published by JAMA in August 2000.[6] What this study did was add up the numbers of medical system-caused deaths. In other words these were deaths that would not have occurred were it not for medical intervention. Additionally these were deaths that were only noted in a hospital setting. The study reported that medical-system-caused deaths accounted for and became the 3rd leading cause of death in the U.S.A.! This is known as iatrogenic death, meaning it would not otherwise have occurred but for medical intervention.

This editorial in JAMA points to the ultimate conflict for an individual and especially for a parent – the main person you rely upon for primary care could also become the main cause of serious harm or injury.

Another observation I have made with respect to studies relates to the environment of the study itself. Medical research is based on environments that scientists have attempted to micro-control. Therapies are developed as a result of these controlled-environment studies. When we apply this therapy to a real-life uncontrolled setting we see all the problems and possibility of real harm related to the power and toxicity found in what is no longer a controlled environment. Thus we begin to see deaths and harmful effects that were not noted in the original study. The JAMA-reported study on iatrogenic deaths told us there is a real inherent factor that is harmful over and above side effects of the therapy itself. These factors found in uncontrolled environments must now be considered when looking at various medical therapies.

An old professor of mine in pharmacology class always said with tongue in cheek that when a new drug was released "we should hurry up and use it while it still had few side effects!" More than 20 years of experience in the pharmaceutical industry, together with the evidence offered in the JAMA report, have taught me the absolute veracity of this statement. I have seen drug after drug taken off the market due to continuous dangerous side effects!! In my 20 years of experience in the nutraceutical (vitamin) industry, the adverse event reporting system has reported no deaths from supplemental vitamins. This has taught me that the relative interest in pharmaceuticals versus nutrients is economic and political, not scientific or health-based. – K.M.

The newspaper headline on January 18, 2001 read "Toronto team unlocks immune system secret." The headline the following day? "Immune system find important but overblown, scientists say."

The initial claim, reporting on a research finding of a genetic protein involved in the body's immune response, claimed that the discovery amounted to a "Holy Grail" that would "thwart cancer, diabetes, heart disease." The next day's about-face said that the discovery had been exaggerated, based on an over-blown press release issued by the researchers.

Which to believe? And what of the reader who only bought the first day's newspaper?

Welcome to the wonderful world of making sense of medical information. Our confusion (and frustration) has only grown with the explosion of information available via the Internet from the comfort of our own homes. There are now thousands of Web sites that range from the most reputable to the downright outrageous.

## Fact, fiction and medical studies

As a parent, you need to separate fact from fiction in obtaining solid, credible information for your child with Down Syndrome. When you're researching a

### DEFINING MOMENT

**In vivo:** in the living organism

**In vitro:** in the laboratory

**Clinical trial:** participants are given some intervention, for example a drug, and then followed up for any outcomes

**Single blind study:** subjects did not know what treatment they were receiving

**Double blind study:** neither subjects nor investigators knew who was receiving what treatment

**Crossover study:** subjects receive both the intervention and control treatments in random order, often with periods without treatment in between

**Randomized controlled study:** participants are chosen at random from among a larger group; each group receives a different intervention (including a placebo) then both groups are studied for outcome. This type of study aims to have identical groups at the outset so that the only difference, the treatment administered, can be attributed for any differences in outcome.

**Case report study:** descriptive reports of a single patient's case history outlining treatments and outcome.

health concern, you want to make sense of medical jargon and scientific studies so you can ask questions of your child's doctors or pharmacist and decide on treatment alternatives. Here are some guidelines and approaches you may find useful.

## Step one: Getting started

- You can learn how to do a medical search by enlisting help from a medical or reference librarian. Some colleges and universities offer adult education courses that cover such topics.
- Purchase a good medical dictionary and a basic anatomy book. This information is also available on the Internet.

## Step two: Who published and who funded?

- It's important that you learn the merits of various scientific journals where studies are published. Some of the more established publications (*The New England Journal of Medicine, The Journal of the American Medical Association, The Lancet*) are well-regarded but at times overly cautious in their approach to reporting. You also need to be aware that these publications have large promotion budgets, so tend to be quoted frequently, often at the expense of smaller but worthy journals.
- One of the most important pieces of information you need to know about a study has to do with potential bias. You need to ask who funded the study, and what financial associations, if any, the investigators or authors have with any company that might gain from study results. An increasing number of publications and medical schools have adopted disclosure policies and conflict-of-interest rules or guidelines. Before you put your faith in the findings of a research study, find out who and what is behind it.

- Be aware that privately-funded research has increased dramatically in recent years. Pharmaceutical companies are the major source of funds for drug research. Even when research is being conducted at an academic institution, private companies may be providing part or all of the funds for the study.

- Many studies receive little or no publication. When research has been corporately funded, the company decides how much distribution and publicity, if any, the study will receive. This ranges from a fullblown multi-media marketing campaign, to relegation to the filing bin without ever seeing the light of day if the corporation isn't happy with the findings.

## Step three: Assessing a study's results

- In addition to a detailed description of methodology and results, most studies include a summary section. This will tell you what the study set out to find, and then what it found. This is usually written in prose so it's easier to understand, and may contain all the essential information that you need.

- Journals with a large public readership such as the *Journal of the American Medical Association (JAMA)* issue editorials and articles that summarize study results and report on issues arising from the study including opposing views. This can be useful in providing much-needed context and analysis.

- Look at the study design. Did it include a large enough number of participants? How were the participants chosen? Who was included and who excluded from participation? Was the study conducted over a long enough period of time?

- When looking at the results of a study, don't forget to assess the human dimensions of its findings. Dr. Thomas Lee, editor of *Journal Watch* and an associate professor of medicine at Harvard Medical School, said that "really important studies talk about something that made people feel better, or made them live longer. An intervention that produces just a difference on a test, but not in the way people feel, is not as important." This refers to the "biological relevance" of a treatment or approach.

## Seven strategies for tracking your child's medical history

Children with Down Syndrome often see their doctor with greater frequency, are referred to specialists more often, and undergo many tests for assessment or monitoring of health problems. The following advice comes from Nutri-Chem's parents based on their personal experience when dealing with doctors and medical tests.

1. Start and maintain a medical file at home. Include names and dates of doctors your child sees, and any prescriptions, tests and procedures your child receives.
2. Obtain copies of your child's medical and test reports for your file.
3. Check the body and summary sections of a report to ensure there are no discrepancies between the information contained in them. If you do find a discrepancy, check it out with your child's doctor. Don't assume that the problem is in your reading of the report – mistakes can and do happen.
4. Doctors often report that the results of a test are "normal." You need to go beyond this statement and ask for a breakdown and explanation including how close your child's results are to the normal range. If borderline, consider having another test later done to monitor changes or trends in your child's levels. For example, the test for thyroid function is an elevation of thyroid stimulating hormone (TSH) even within the normal range. Many physicians advocate treating an elevated TSH within the normal range when symptoms support the treatment. A child with Down Syndrome who is

obese and lethargic with a TSH in the upper range of normal, may be considered a candidate for thyroid hormone.

5. Systems in our bodies connect to other systems. Be sure to find out what implications there are for any abnormal results on other systems and functions in the body.

6. Consider keeping a journal that includes a summary of the information in your child's home medical file. This can be as simple as a small, spiral-bound notebook that you can carry with you at all times. This is extremely useful in emergencies, but also for visits to specialists who may ask you questions about your child's medical history.

7. Finally, make sure you get all your questions answered after your child has had a test or procedure. You may consider asking someone to accompany you for those times when emotional upset can cloud your ability to hear or concentrate on what you are being told. Keep a written list of your questions, and record the answers. Some parents also tape record, with the doctor's knowledge, certain vital meetings for further reference.

# Closing comments from Kent:

*WHAT ARE PARENTS TO DO?*

*The main causes of death based on the JAMA study were: drug errors (wrong drug and wrong dose) and adverse effects of prescribed drugs. Additionally, there is always a danger factor with any drug or surgical intervention above and beyond the inherent risk of the drug or procedure itself. With this in mind you must be your own best advocate for yourself or your child. My advice? It would seem prudent to have on your side a pharmacist who is the drug expert and someone you feel is working on your behalf and not on behalf of a drug company or physician. You should feel free to ask or pay for an independent evaluation of any drug therapy offered to you or your child.*

*I now routinely ask the patients with whom I consult to bring in their lab results for me to review. There have been countless times when patients tell me that they have been told their results are one thing when in fact the interpretation is wrong. Very few people are able to read and understand lab results. Therefore, my last piece of advice is that if you are unable to find a professional you are confident can give you expert advice on your child's drug therapy, or that you are confident fully understands the lab results, you should seek out other medical resources, such as those found at Nutri-Chem. – K.M.*

# Endnotes

1. "Influence of vitamin A nutriture on the immune response: findings in children with Down's syndrome." (1978) *International Journal of Vitamin and Nutrition Research.* 48(2):188-216

2. Meydani, S., et al. (1997) "Vitamin E supplementation and in vivo immune response in healthy elderly subjects." *Journal of the American Medical Association* 277: 1380-86

3. D'Souza, R.M., D'Souza, R. (2002) "Vitamin A for treating measles in children." *Cochrane Database Syst* Rev. 1: CD001479

4. Arrieta A.C., et al. (1992) "Vitamin A levels in children with measles in Long Beach, California." *Journal of Pediatrics.* 121(1):75-8

5. Stephens D., et al "Subclinical vitamin A deficiency: a potentially unrecognized problem in the United States." (1996) *Pediatric Nursing.* 22(5):377-89, 456

6. Barbara Starfield, (2000) "Is US Health Really the Best in the World?" *Journal of the American Medical Association* 284: 483-5

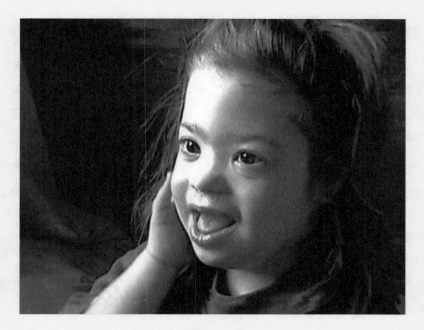

**EMILY JANAK**

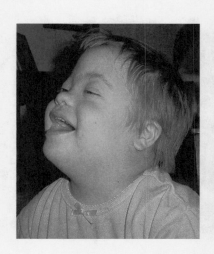

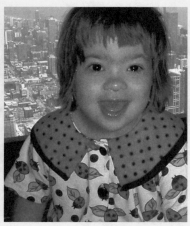

# CHAPTER 12

# ONE MOTHER'S STORY

*WE OFTEN THINK THAT RESEARCH AND INQUIRY IS MOTIVATED BY SOME HIGHER SCIENTIFIC PURPOSE. The reality is often quite different. Research and scientific activity is driven by parents' insistence on some action on behalf of their children. Nothing illustrates this more clearly that the case of Laurette Janak. Her consistent, intelligent and passionate approach to the medical threats to her child, coupled with Laurette's concern for all children, inspired many health professionals, including myself, to reach for deeper levels of understanding where Down Syndrome is concerned.*

*As I look back on my involvement with Laurette and her daughter Emily, it seems that the only time she was on the receiving end of information was the first time we met. From then on, I was constantly overwhelmed with the volume of information Laurette sent my way. It would take me some time to digest the information and place it into the context of what was then known about Down Syndrome, before I could adequately convey these new findings to other parents. Because of my own experience, I can appreciate how daunting it was for the average medical doctor to be confronted by the depth and volume of Laurette's knowledge.*

## WHAT WILL I LEARN?

▸ How a life-saving drug could be deadly.

▸ What the SAM cycle means to your child's health.

▸ A mother's advice on getting good medical care for your child.

*For her part, Laurette is constantly frustrated by the lack of understanding around her. Think about it – the odds of any health professional cracking open a biochemistry textbook are about the same as them making a medical house call. This does not mean that physicians lack compassion. It does, however, explain a physician's comfort level in following the status quo when using an alternative means deciphering literally volumes of new information.*

*Physicians and other health professionals need to simplify things. Much of this chapter involves understanding complex and new information. It will discuss folic acid and its relationship to neural tube defects causing a debilitating disorder with significant costs to the child affected, the family and society itself. We cannot be discouraged from understanding the importance of the systems discussed in this chapter. We owe it to children now and those yet born to find safer non-toxic treatments for the prevention and treatment of disease in Down Syndrome.*

*I dedicate this chapter to Emily and Laurette Janak. – K.M.*

---

When Laurette J.'s mother-in-law called her in Chicago in May, 1995, she delivered the kind of good news any aunt loves to hear: Laurette had a newborn niece. A second call came fifteen minutes later, saying that the family's excitement had turned to dismay – the baby had Down Syndrome.

Soon after, Laurette learned that her sister-in-law had decided to put her daughter up for adoption and baby Emily would be going home from hospital with her grandmother for the time being. "Emily's mother had a two-year-old at home," Laurette recalls. "She was under a great deal of emotional stress at the time. My sister-in-law wanted the best for her baby, and she believed she could not give that to her."

For Laurette, it was eerily reminiscent of a dream she'd had. In it, she could see a group of people in the distance, gathered around a baby's crib. They were excited, but as Laurette moved closer, she could see the looks on their faces turn from joy to sadness. When the phone calls came announcing Emily's birth, Laurette remembered the dream, and knew her prayer for a second child had been answered.

"I had lived my whole life, ever since I was a little girl, wanting to be a mom," says Laurette. In her early twenties, this had looked impossible as doctors told Laurette she would likely never have children, even going so far as to recommend she have a hysterectomy. Devastated at this news, but determined to have a child, Laurette turned to holistic and nutritional therapies. After one miscarriage, her son Steven was born in 1985, but her dream of more children wasn't realized as several more miscarriages followed Steven's birth.

With her sister-in-law's blessing, Laurette and her husband, Ray, traveled to Buffalo, New York, their hometown, and welcomed Emily as their daughter. "I didn't think about her Down Syndrome," says Laurette. "I just thought of Emily as a child to love. When I look back on it now, I remember thinking that I was smart enough to handle any challenges that Emily's Down Syndrome could present. I didn't know then that Emily would become my teacher and I would learn powerful lessons from her."

When Laurette brought six-week-old Emily home for the first time, she was focused only on getting right to work loving her daughter and giving her the best possible start in life. What she didn't know then was that her much-loved little girl would face a life-and-death battle with cancer before her fourth birthday and a brain injury from the drug treatments that were needed to cure her leukemia.

## The 'rule of two'

Laurette had heard about vitamin therapies for babies and young children with Down Syndrome. She was "absolutely convinced" that nutritional therapies had enabled her to avoid a hysterectomy and become pregnant with Steven. So it was natural that she wanted to start Emily on vitamins right away. Research led her to Kent MacLeod at Nutri-Chem.

"The first time I called him, we spoke for 45 minutes. I had a lot of questions, and Kent was patient in answering them. I did a lot of research and found there was nothing that could hurt Emily in Nutri-Chem's MSB nutritional supplements, so she started on MSB at three months of age. I felt good about that. Then I learned about individualized testing and it was something I wanted to have done. I would send the lab results to Nutri-Chem, and they would adjust Emily's formula and I felt good about that."

At three months of age, Emily had her first immunization vaccine. "My healthy daughter started to get sick – real sick. I asked the doctors if it could have anything to do with the immunization. Although Emily was sick enough to be hospitalized for a week, the doctors said that it had nothing to do with her vaccination. I believed them, but three months later she had her second vaccination and got sick again."

Laurette developed her rule of two: if you go back a second time with something wrong and you're told that nothing's wrong, it's time to take action. Knowing that children with Down Syndrome have weaker immune systems and believing that the immunizations had further weakened Emily's, Laurette told the doctors "That's it – no more immunizations."

For some time, Laurette had been taking Emily every six months to the Institute for the Achievement of Human Potential in Philadelphia. Here, parents are instructed in home-based programs aimed at improving their children's health, including physical therapy and nutrition. They also work with neurologists and other medical staff, and biochemists who conduct blood and urine analysis. Laurette had tests done on Emily at an independent laboratory and sent the results to Nutri-Chem so they could tailor her daughter's nutritional supplements based on needs identified by the testing.

Emily was healthy and developing well, but in February of 1998 as she approached her third birthday, her blood test revealed a dramatically elevated MCV (mean corpuscular volume) level. In an average three-year-old, a normal MCV level, which is age-related, is approximately 85. For a three-year-old with Down Syndrome the level jumps to an average of 90. Emily's MCV reading was an alarming 98. This was a red flag to the Philadelphia doctors, indicating that Emily had macrocytosis, an increase in the size of red blood cells caused by disrupted DNA synthesis. Because of the connection between macrocytosis and disturbances in the folate cycle common in Down Syndrome, the doctors in Philadelphia recommended that Emily have B12 injections. Laurette took this prescription to Emily's doctor in Buffalo who refused to give the B12 injections because tests showed Emily's levels of B12 and folate were not insufficient. In fact, they were elevated and in the case of B12, extremely high.

## Cause for concern

Caught between the advice of doctors at the Institute in Philadelphia, and her local doctor's refusal to act on this advice, Laurette swung into action. Like most parents of children with Down Syndrome, she had been researching and learning about the genetic disorder that affected her daughter. She'd always been someone who had to know how and why things happened the way they did. Now she became a one-woman research institute, determined to find an answer to what it meant to have such an elevated MCV level. What she learned increased her concern about Emily's health to the point of alarm.

"I read and read and read about macrocytosis and the folate cycle. I learned about folate trapping – the folate was there, but it couldn't be used." Because of the link between folate deficiencies and DNA alterations, Laurette became concerned about the possibility that Emily would develop cancer.

As September approached, Emily was due to start school and was required to have her immunization updated. Laurette was concerned based on past experience that it had weakened Emily's immune system, but feeling her daughter was basically well she agreed to the vaccination. Once again, Emily became sick. And as Laurette continued to research the links between folate, DNA and cancer, she became frightened.

# A parent's nightmare

In November, Laurette opened Emily's diaper and found it soaked in blood. She rushed her to the hospital. Tests were conducted and on December 22, 1998, Emily J. was diagnosed with acute lymphocytic leukemia. By this time, Laurette understood what was happening in Down Syndrome that affected two important cycles related to DNA: the folate cycle and the SAM cycle. She knew that Emily's folate was "trapped" and she was functionally deficient in folate. She knew that methionine synthase activity, already low in children with Down Syndrome, was even lower in Emily. She also knew that methotrexate, the chemotherapy drug doctors were planning to use to treat Emily's leukemia, shuts down folate and knocks out methionine synthase. Laurette questioned the chemotherapy protocol that the doctors were proposing to use on Emily and her first chemo dosage was reduced by half. Seeing no adverse reaction in Emily, the doctors then dismissed Laurette's concerns and future doses were at 100% levels. Laurette was told the protocol had a 70% success rate.

"My daughter had an extra sensitivity to methotrexate, but no one looked at why. One of the reasons why is the overexpression of cystathione beta synthase (CBS) found on the 21st chromosome which is pulling homocysteine away and affecting methionine synthase levels. I said be careful because methotrexate affects a line of chemistry that's already affected in Down Syndrome. Children with Down Syndrome have low SAM levels to begin with, and Emily's were lower than most. They were going to give her a drug that would make her status worse. SAM does a lot of things in the body and one of the places where it is most important is in the brain, in neurotransmitter production and in maintenance of the myelin sheath that protects nerve cells. That's what happened to Emily – the myelin sheath was damaged, and her brain and spinal chord sustained injury."

At the time of Emily's leukemia diagnosis in December, her CAT scan had been completely normal. Within three weeks after starting chemotherapy treatment, she had lost her speech and fine motor skills, and could no longer walk. She sat in her crib, cross-eyed, grinding her teeth, rocking back and forth, and pounding her head against the side. After a second CAT scan in March, Laurette insisted that an MRI be performed. This was done in April, 1999, and the result was a diagnosis of chemo-related brain injury called leukoencephalopathy, a condition normally seen only after a year or more of chemotherapy treatments. Laurette also insisted on a spinal MRI which showed Emily had chemo-related spinal chord damage called leukomalasia.

## 'Find another way'

Facing two more years of chemotherapy, Laurette grew desperate and insisted that another chemo protocol be found. Until the doctors figured out another approach, Emily would have no further treatments.

The doctors investigated alternate forms of treatment, and offered a drug protocol which involved lower dosages of methotrexate administered continuously instead of every three weeks as with the previous protocol. An added bonus of this approach was a higher success rate, 75% instead of the previous 70%. "This is a significant difference if your child is among the 5%," Laurette says.

## Forming a better response

Folic acid is the synthetic form of folate commonly added to breads, pastas and vitamins. It undergoes several steps as the body converts it into a functional form for its use. Folinic acid is a preferable supplement for children with Down Syndrome who have a functional folate deficiency. Folinic acid appears to be a more metabolically active form of folate, able to bypass some of the steps required to make it available for DNA synthesis.

After two weeks without chemo, Emily resumed treatment.

Methotrexate is an anti-folate drug. Fast-dividing cancer cells need DNA material to keep reproducing. If you turn off the folate cycle, you turn off the raw materials needed for producing DNA and the cell dies. Because of the way the SAM cycle functions in children with Down Syndrome, while the anti-folate was attacking Emily's cancer cells it was also causing rapid brain deterioration in Emily. Laurette became determined to find a way to provide Emily with a folate alternative without interfering with the efficacy of her anti-folate cancer drug.

Laurette studied children born with genetic defects in enzymes called "inborn errors of metabolism." She found that the body has a secondary enzyme called Betaine Homocysteine Methyl Transferase (BHMT) which can be utilized along a separate pathway in the SAM cycle to recycle more of the homocysteine and raise the levels of methionine, thus protecting the myelin sheath of brain cells without having to use folate or $B_{12}$.

# Unravelling the science

Laurette began giving Emily a supplement called Tri Methyl Glycine (TMG), a form of betaine. Emily's SAM cycle levels were determined with a test called a Thiol Panel. It gives what Laurette calls a moving picture of a dynamic cycle, not just a static number which results from a typical folate count. After Emily was given the TMG supplement, her Thiol Panel showed that more of the homocysteine was being converted to methionine without folate or B12. Enough of the SAM was getting to Emily's brain cells and the myelin sheath was being rebuilt. Each MRI since has shown an improvement and at this point in time the results have returned to what is termed "near-normal." Emily's tremors are gone, her speech is returning, she's walking and back in school. And while she still has neurological and gastrointestinal problems from the chemotherapy and a weakened immune system, Emily has finished her treatments and her latest bone marrow test was clear. Her cancer is in remission.

Another result of Emily's chemotherapy was the onset of osteopenia (loss of bone mass sometimes known as demineralization) which resulted in four separate fractures during one year of her treatment. Steroids included as part of her chemotherapy had caused Emily's calcium and vitamin D levels to drop to dangerously low levels. "This effect of treatment is known, yet Emily's levels were never checked and my daughter had to endure pain and suffering from broken bones which could have been prevented with nutritional intervention," Laurette says.

Throughout Emily's cancer treatments, she remained on her customized MSB supplement. Because of the need to remove folate with the cancer drugs to slow down DNA formation in the cancer cells, it was removed from her MSB as well. Laurette's goal was to give Emily's immune system extra support, so she had Nutri-Chem increase the immune-boosting nutrients such as vitamin E and co-enzyme Q10, as well as lipoic acid. Since chemotherapy can create free radicals, Emily's MSB formula was modified during that period to increase the antioxidants. When Emily's osteopenia was diagnosed, the hospital supplied separate supplements of additional calcium and vitamin D.

"There were many, many, many times when Emily could or would not eat during her cancer treatments. The hospital had no problem with that as long as she was taking her cancer drugs. I felt that the vitamin supplements were giving my daughter at least a basic level of nutrition that she wasn't getting from food. Basically, I look on her MSB supplements as an inexpensive insurance policy."

## A mother's words

Here's what Laurette says today about her daughter's ordeal: "I believe that when you don't know something and you don't act, that's ignorance. When you know something and you don't act, that's negligence. The relationship between Down Syndrome and cancer or Autism exists, and we need to find out why.

"Cancer happens because there's a predisposition in a person, and then something happens that acts as a trigger. This can be something in the person's lifestyle such as smoking or high levels of stress. It can be something in the external environment such as chemical pollution. In the case of Down Syndrome, there's a pre-existing immune system problem. There is also a metabolic disturbance in two very important cycles, the folate cycle and the SAM cycle, related to synthesis and repair of DNA which becomes altered in cases of cancer.

"We need to look at the similarities between Down Syndrome and Autism, and ask why? Can we avert these diseases if we intervene sufficiently to eliminate the predisposing factors? What role does the mercury in immunization vaccines play as a trigger in disease? These are questions that need to be answered. I am driven to find out why things happen and what can be done to change the outcome so that my daughter's pain and suffering are not in vain."

## Laurette's advice to parents

From her experience with Emily, and her own research, Laurette offers the following advice:

- Have your child screened yearly for thyroid and have a CBC (Complete Blood Count) done at the same time. The test should be done and assessed by a hemotologist. Abnormally high MCV levels are a red-flag warning that something's wrong and should not be ignored. Possible causes are kidney, liver or thyroid problems, or a problem with folate and vitamin $B_{12}$ in the SAM/folate cycles. Underactive thyroid or pernicious anemia are associated with higher incidences of leukemia.

- Have your child's immune system levels checked before giving immunizations. Mercury preservatives in vaccines can further suppress the immune system and blood platelets. Intestinal bleeding and rashes are signs of mercury poisoning. If you choose to have your child immunized, be sure you are providing optimal support for her immune system.

- If your child is diagnosed with leukemia, have an endocrinologist monitor your child throughout to prevent osteopenia.

- If your child says "it hurts to walk," have it checked out. This is a common complaint of children who later develop leukemia because a high percentage of these children already have bone metabolism disruptions at the time of cancer diagnosis

- If your child is on steroids, have their calcium and vitamin D levels checked and supplement if the levels are low.

- Learn how to read medical studies. One of the best web sites I have found is pubmed (www.ncbi.nlm.nih.gov/pubmed). It links to the National Library of Medicine's complete listing of international journals and their study abstracts, and is a free service. Often the "review" articles are the easiest to understand since they're often written by graduate students and include summaries of articles. You can use Medscape to search topics, and sign up for weekly e-mail updates on specific subjects. These are often in the form of press releases, so they're written in plain language and easy to understand.

- Get yourself two essential reference books: a good medical dictionary, and a college anatomy/physiology book. Summer yard sales are a great place to pick these up at low cost.

- Perhaps most important of all is not to be intimidated because you don't know the language of science. The only way to know is to get in there with both feet and start. It's like learning another language. At first you can't understand what people are talking about, but through exposure and trial and error, you start to learn the basics. Eventually, you can speak the language at least enough to ask important questions. When you don't understand the answers you're given, ask the medical professional two questions: "What does this mean?" and "How will this affect my child?"

# The SAM cycle

## Say hello to SAM

One of the best ways to understand the SAM cycle and its role as a major methyl group donor (more on this later), is to think of it as the finishing carpenter of a newly-constructed house. After the foundation is laid, the walls are up, and the roof is on, the house looks complete. But it's the work of the finishing carpenter to attach handles on the doors to allow you to move around inside the house.

The SAM cycle, which requires folic acid and vitamin B12 to work, is a cycle involving a group of amino acids and amino acid derivatives. It transports methyl groups (called attaching groups) to get them where they're needed – from one room in the house to another. It has a critical role in DNA methylation to detoxify chemicals in the body and is needed as a precursor for production of neurotransmitters and maintenance of the myelin sheath that protects nerve cells. A methyl group (three units of hydrogen combined with one unit of carbon) is essential for the formation of DNA which reproduces itself each time a cell divides. Methyl groups are obtained common dietary components such as amino acids (serine, glycine, methionine), and choline which comes from the breakdown of a specific type of fat.

If you look at the SAM cycle diagram, you see the flow of amino aciDown Syndrome and how they are converted by contact with specific enzymes. The amino acid homocysteine travels in two directions, both of which are important. In one direction, homocysteine is being drawn toward conversion into glutathione, the "anti-aging" protein that protects cells. On its journey, it encounters CBS (cystathionine-beta synthase), a gene found on the 21st chromosome with coding for production of the CBS protein. Along its second pathway, homocysteine interacts with the methionine synthase (MS) enzyme and vitamin B12 on its way to conversion into methionine (essential for DNA). Folate plays a key role by transferring its methyl group to the B12 at this point in the cycle so the folate can become functionally active with the homocysteine as it regenerates methionine.

# Sam Cycle

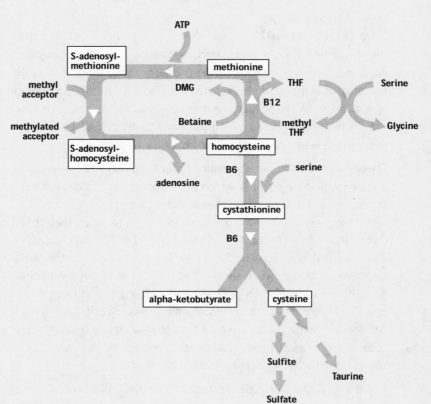

## Why is SAM important in Down Syndrome?

In Down Syndrome, CBS (found on the 21st chromosome) is elevated, affecting the amount of homocysteine travelling along its two pathways.[1, 2, 3] If you think of the CBS as a paper cup with two holes in the bottom, there is a third hole in the cup of someone with Down Syndrome. More of the homocysteine is draining through that extra hole, leaving less homocysteine to travel along its other path toward methionine regeneration.

At the point in the cycle where folate is involved, it "pools" because it is unable to transfer its methyl group to the homocysteine. This is known as the methyl-folate trap or functional folate deficiency because despite sufficient levels of folate, it can't be used to regenerate sufficient methionine for the production of SAM. If there is insufficient folate to carry the methyl groups, DNA synthesis is affected. If DNA is not being made, your cells cannot divide.

These effects are most apparent first in the most rapidly-dividing cells, the red cell precursors in bone marrow. The result is that the red blood cells keep getting bigger. This phenomenon is called macrocytosis, (meaning big), evidence of which will be found in high MCV (mean corpuscular volume) measured by MCB levels in a Complete Blood Count (CBC) test. Although macrocytosis is well documented in Down Syndrome, it has perplexed researchers because serum folate as measured in standard blood tests is usually normal.[4, 5, 6, 7] It is now thought that if a functional folate deficiency is present, this might account for the macrocytosis.

An article in *Pediatric Research* in December 1985 observed the death of a three-and-a-half-year-old girl due to a folic acid deficiency.[8] This girl had normal blood folic acid and almost no methyl THF (folinic

> ## DEFINING MOMENT
>
> **Anemia:** Insufficient number of red blood cells or hemoglobin in blood.
>
> **Hemoglobin:** Red pigment in blood that combines with oxygen to produce cellular energy
>
> **S-adenosylmethionine (SAM):** the active methyl donor that is a vital part of countless metabolic reactions throughout the body
>
> **The SAM cycle:** a cycle that helps transport methylgroups organisms
>
> **Methyl group:** One unit of carbon (basic element from which all organic matter is created) combined with three units of hydrogen; essential in production of DNA

## DEFINING MOMENT

**DNA (deoxyribonucleic acid):** chemical inside cell nucleus carrying genetic instructions for production of living organisms (DNA in genes is constantly mutating and being repaired)

**Mean corpuscular volume (MCV):** test that measures macrocytosis

**Macrocytosis:** Increase in red blood cell size due to inability to divide because DNA synthesis has been disturbed

**Cystathionine-beta synthase (CBS):** gene located on the 21st chromosome with coding for production of the CBS protein which acts as an enzyme in chain reaction conversion of amino acid in Down Syndrome: homocysteine to cystathionine to cysteine, a precursor to glutathione (necessary to protect liver and brain from toxic substances)

**Homocysteine:** amino acid made from methionine that in turn converts into other amino acids

**Amino acids:** organic substances that make proteins

**Enzymes:** biological substances made up of proteins that act as catalysts

**Folate:** functions as a single carbon donor in synthesis of DNA; needed for production of red blood cells, tissue growth and cell function

**Folic Acid:** synthetic form of folate found in supplements or added to foods

acid), which is the active form of folic acid. This occurrence has been applied on a broader and more universal scale because it has been shown that as much as 30% of the population may have a genetically altered ability to form active folic acid. (folinic acid). This creates a significantly enhanced requirement of folic acid. This has been implied in the risk of neural tube defects, colorectal cancer, and even in the very cause of Down Syndrome.[9] It is important to note that in these mutations that normal serum levels of B12 and folic acid can occur but essentially there can be a significant active folic acid deficiency. This can be circumvented by the use of folinic acid. Jill James demonstrated that levels of homocysteine, methionine, S-Adenosyl-methionine and S-Adenosyl-homocysteine were all significantly decreased in children with Down Syndrome.[10] These effects will also aggravate or contribute to potential folic acid and B12 deficiency.

Gluthione is also depressed in Down Syndrome. It has been shown experimentally that glutathione depletion causes an extensive overutilization and lowering of methionine, which causes an alteration in DNA methylation.[11]

# The Anemia Connection

Anemia is a condition where blood has reduced levels of red blood cells or of hemoglobin which is needed for oxygen to get from your lungs to cells throughout your body so that those cells can produce energy. This means your body will be tired, and your brain duller because it is deprived of energy-producing oxygen. Anemia also affects how well your body's cells can build and repair themselves.

There are several different types of anemia, with different causes. Nutritionally, vitamin B12 and folate deficiencies are important because insufficient vitamin B12 leads to a secondary folate deficiency where the folate gets trapped and can't do its job. And remember, even if you have enough folate in your system, if the body has malfunctioned you can't use the folate that is there. It's like having a full tank of gas but no fuel line to get it to the engine. The result is a type of anemia referred to as pernicious anemia.

Increased folate in the diet can treat this form of anemia, however if vitamin B12 is still lacking, the additional folate can mask the B12 deficiency. If left untreated, this can lead to permanent nerve damage and eventual paralysis. Supplements of folic acid, therefore, need to also contain vitamin B12.

We know that B12 is essential for SAM cycle function and it will increase methionine synthase activity. In addition to the benefits on blood and nerve, B12 will also improve the immune system by increasing T-lymphocyctes and natural killer cells.[12]

# Folic acid and thyroid function

Thyroid disfunction affects as many as 25% of children with Down Syndrome. Folic acid is important in Down Syndrome because it has been shown to improve thyroid function.[13] Infants with Down Syndrome receiving supplemental folic acid had significantly less thyroid dysfunction.

How is thyroid function connected to folic acid? These are but a few of many proven ways:

- hypothyroidism decreases hepatic levels of enzyme involved in the remethylation pathway of homocysteine;[14]

- folate mediated incorporation of histidine into DNA is influenced by thyroid;[15]

- MTHFR levels are decreased in hypothyroidism.[15]

## Acetylcholine and the SAM cycle

Acetylcholine is an essential neuro transmitter and is crucial for the proper function of the parasympathetic nervous system, which effects every part of the body. Acetylcholine deficiency has been show in Down Syndrome[16] and has been demonstrated by a marked hypersensitivity to atropine in Down Syndrome.

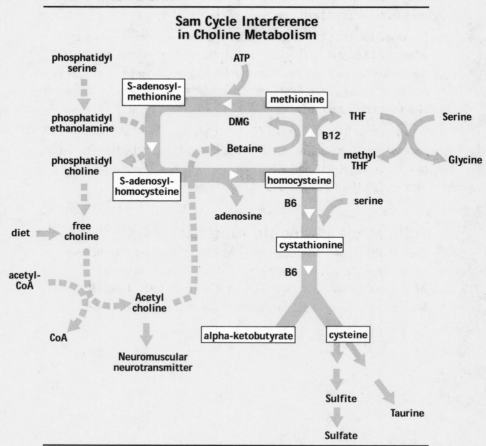

**Sam Cycle Interference in Choline Metabolism**

In the diagram, we see that SAM depletion will cause a depletion of in vivo synthesis of acetylcholine. In addition, choline depletion can be caused by a depleted SAM cycle as shown in the diagram. Furthermore, choline can be used as a source of methyl groups for the SAM cycle, through its conversion to betaine. So choline depletion and disturbance is intimately connected to the SAM cycle.

## Brain development and choline

The neo-natal requirement for choline in brain development may create a folic acid deficiency in gestation. Depleting dietary choline causes enduring adverse effects in the brain.[17] Children administered with choline have shown improvements to verbal and visual memory.[18] Deficits of enzyme-forming acetylcholine were found in the brains of both Down Syndrome and Alzheimer's patients.[19]

This same enzyme was studied in episodic apnea, which is common in Down Syndrome. In one study, a disturbance of this enzyme-forming acetylcholine (choline acetyltransfurace) caused a myasthenic syndrome associated with episodic apnea in humans.[20] This is particularly interesting in Down Syndrome as there is a much higher incidence of episodic apnea. Again, based on this work an impairment of this enzyme would result in a deficiency of acetylcholine. This enzyme is dependent on adequate levels of SAM.

The enzyme choline acetyltransfurace requires acetyl co A to function. Acetyle co A function is dependent on pantothenic acid, cysteine and carnitine for its formation.

Choline is present as phospholipids in foods such as eggs, liver and soybeans, and as free choline in certain vegetables such as cauliflower.

Betaine is present in some foods such as beets.

Deficiency seems to increase an enzyme called alanine aminotransferase which would deplete alanine and ketoglutarate. Requirements of choline, as determined by food and nutrition boards, are from 100 mg (newborn infants) to 500 mg per day (adults).

## So what does this mean?

First of all, aceylcholine is proven to be low in Down Syndrome. It is essential for proper function and development of the brain and other organs. Its formation and regulation is intimately tied to the methylation cycle and levels of folic acid. Supplementing with choline has shown to have some benefits in focus and attention with no adverse effects. Extra choline will improve methylation and active folic acid and B12 in the SAM cycle.

## The cancer connection

Collectively, the evidence from the study of disease in animals and humans strongly suggests that folate status modulates the risk of developing cancers in selected tissue. Folate depletion appears to enhance cancers whereas folate supplementation appears to convey a protective effect.[21]

Any factor – environmental, dietary or genetics – which interferes with folic acid metabolism will increase risk of cancer. One of the cancers which the evidence is most notable in is colorectal cancer.[16] The dramatically enhanced rates of leukemia in Down Syndrome may have its origins in this problem as well. It is confusing that the treatment for this leukemia is an antifolate drug called methotrexate. It has been shown that children with Down Syndrome are much more sensitive to the adverse effects of methotrexate, as Laurette discovered with Emily. This is to be expected, given that they are far more likely to be folic-acid deficient. Therefore, if they take an antifolate drug, it is likely that they will suffer more side effects, as Emily did. When children with Down Syndrome are subjected to treatments using the drug methotrexate, it is important to use folinic acid to rescue the body from the severe side effects of folic acid depletion. The other name for this folinic acid is leucovorin. Incidentally, leucovorin is also used in the basic chemotherapy protocol for colorectal cancer.

Folic acid is being routinely added to many foods you purchase in grocery stores because governments are recognizing the importance of this supplement in disease prevention.

# Closing comments from Kent:

*It is my experience that the population at large including the medical profession, is not aware of the significance of folic acid and SAM cycle in disease prevention. If we don't believe or understand the importance of using folic acid itself, how are we to understand the workings of the folic acid cycle, the SAM cycle and their inter-relationships? The SAM cycle and methylation cycle have many key pieces necessary for their functioning – folic acid, B6, B12, choline, glutathione, zinc, acetyl co A,and many others. The gross problems associated with these key elements on disease prevention are just beginning to be understood and utilized on the population as a whole. The subtle biochemical individualities and variations and additional requirements caused by the Down Syndrome genetic makeup are even more essential for disease prevention in Down Syndrome. – K.M.*

# Endnotes

1. Chadefaux, B., et al. (1985) "Cystathionine beta-synthase: gene dosage effect in trisomy 21." *Biochemistry and Biophysical Research Communications* 128: 40-44.

2. Chadefaux, B., et al. (1988) "Is absence of atheroma in Down syndrome due to decreased homocysteine levels?" *Lancet* 1: 741.

3. Pogribna, M., et al (2001) "Homocysteine metabolism in children with Down syndrome: in vitro modulation." *American Journal of Human Genetics.* 69(1): 88-95.

4. David, O., et al. (1996) "Hematological studies in children with Down syndrome." *Pediatric Hematology and Oncology.* 13(3): 271-5.

5. Roizen N.J., Amarose, A.P. (1993) "Hematologic abnormalities in children with Down syndrome." *American Journal of Medical Genetics.* 46(5): 510-2.

6. Wachtel T.J., Pueschel, S.M. (1991) "Macrocytosis in Down syndrome." *American Journal of Mental Retardation.* 95(4): 417-20.

7. Gericke, G.S., et al. (1977) "Leucocyte ultrastructure and folate metabolism in Down's syndrome." *South African Medical Journal.* 51(12): 369-74

8. Baumgartner, E.R., et al. (1985) "Comparison of folic acid coenzyme distribution patterns in patients with methylenetetrahydrofolate reductase and methionine synthase deficiencies." *Pediatric Research.* 19(12): 1288-92

9. Choi, S.-W., and Mason, J. (2000) "Folate and Carcinogenesis." *Journal of Nutrition* 130: 129-32.

10. Pogribna, M., et al. (2001) "Homocysteine metabolism in children with Down syndrome: in vitro modulation." *American Journal of Human Genetics* 69(1): 88-95

11. Lertratanangkoon, K., et al. (1997) "Alterations of DNA methylation by glutathione depletion." *Cancer Letters* 120(2): 149-156.

12. Tamura, J., et al. (1999) "Immunomodulation by vitamin B12: augmentation of CD8+ T lymphocytes and natural killer (NK) cell activity in vitamin B12-deficient patients by methyl-B12 treatment." *Clinical and Experimental Immunology.* 116(1): 28-32.

13. Peeters, M. (1995) "Elevated TSH levels in young children with Down syndrome: beneficial effects of supplemental folic acid." *Pediatric Rev. Commun* 8: 97-103

14. Catargi B., et al. (1999) "Homocysteine, hypothyroidism, and effect of thyroid hormone replacement." *Thyroid.* 9(12):1163-6.

15. Nair, C.P., et al. "(1994) Folate-mediated incorporation of ring-2-carbon of histidine into nucleic acids: influence of thyroid hormone." *Metabolism* 43(12): 1575-8.

16. Godridge, H., et al. (1987) "Alzheimer-like neurotransmitter deficits in adult Down's syndrome brain tissue." *Journal of Neurology, Neurosurgery and Psychiatry* 50(6): 775-8.

17. Montoya, D.A.C., et al.(2000). "Prenatal choline exposure alters hippocampal responsiveness to cholinergic stimulation in adulthood." *Developmental Brain Research* 123(1): 25-32.

18. Buchman, A.L., et al. (2001) "Verbal and visual memory improve after choline supplementation in long-term total parenteral nutrition: A pilot study." *Journal of Parenteral and Enteral Nutrition* 25: 30-5.

19. Schneider, C., et al. (1997) "Similar deficits of central histaminergic system in patients with Down syndrome and Alzheimer disease." *Neuroscience Letters* 222(3): 183-6.

20. Ohno, K., et al. (2001) "Choline acetyltransferase mutations cause myasthenic syndrome associated with episodic apnea in humans." *Proceedings of the National Academy of Sciences USA* 89(4): 2017-2022.

21. Choi, S.-W., and Mason, J. (2000) "Folate and Carcinogenesis." *Journal of Nutrition* 130: 129-32.

# SECTION 5
# WHAT YOU CAN DO

## CHAPTER 13
### How Nutri-Chem Can Help

## CHAPTER 14
### Research for Tomorrow

# CADE'S STORY

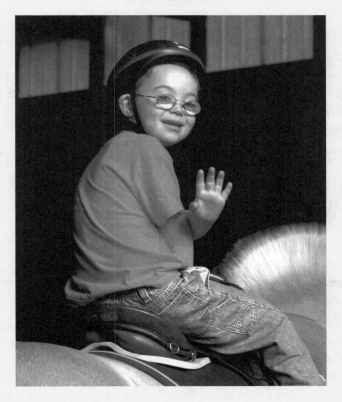

When Kim Holden found the source of her infant son's illness five years ago, it was the route to better health for her as well. Food additives in Kim's breast milk were causing baby Cade's continuous vomiting and recurring pneumonia. They were also the reason Kim had fuzzy thinking, no energy, was tired all the time and chronically underweight. "My symptoms went away as soon as I removed the food additives," says Kim. "And not only did Cade stop throwing up, his ability to sign (communicate) just took off. He had 150 signs before he started talking."

Kim was told six weeks before Cade was born that he had Down Syndrome. He arrived several weeks early, and needed stomach surgery the day after his birth. While in the hospital, Cade's father ran into a friend who practiced acupressure. "She said 'You absolutely have to get these vitamins for the baby'," Kim recalls. "I do a lot of alternative stuff, so I was very open to the idea because the one thing I had been told about kids with Down Syndrome is that they get sick all the time. I dragged my feet a little because Nutri-Chem was in Canada."

A dinner engagement sparked Kim to act. "There was a 14-year-old with Down Syndrome at the dinner," she says. "He had such terrible upper respiratory infection.It was too much for me to see. We left there and I said 'I'm going to call about the vitamins right away'. We started Cade on them one week later."

With the exception of Cade's reaction to food additives, he's been a healthy little boy. Cataracts at birth have left him legally blind and he does have ear tubes for fluid buildup. But he has never developed the asthma that doctors predicted he would and Kim says he's had only two colds in five years.

"I know the supplements work for Cade," his mother says, "because last summer I cut his dosage to every second day after finding that his urine had become very yellow. Within two weeks, his behaviour changed – from a very social little boy, to one who would leave a group of people he knew, lie down in his room by himself, and suck his finger. It took me a couple of days to notice, and I wondered if it was because I had reduced his vitamins. As soon as I put him back on his daily dose of vitamins, the behavioural changes stopped."

As well as removing foods with chemical additives, Kim has eliminated wheat and dairy from Cade's diet. "Recently we were out to eat, and I said, 'Oh, let him have some pancakes'. He developed an upper respiratory infection right away."

Cade is "really into people," his mother says, and loves swimming and putting on plays with his sister, seven-year-old Savannah.

"I can't ever imagine Cade not having MSB," his mother says. "We feel the vitamins have made a difference in his life and in ours."

# CHAPTER 13

# HOW NUTRI-CHEM CAN HELP

*THE LANDSCAPE OF NUTRITION AND DOWN SYNDROME IS LITTERED WITH CONTRADICTION AND CONTROVERSY. As a chemist, it was obvious to me that the clinical laboratory was the place to clear up some of the ignorance and debate surrounding Down Syndrome.*

The simplicity underlying the controversy and arguments that go around in circles is illustrated by looking at one nutrient: iron. Without testing, we have groups that claim iron is bad for you. On the other hand, iron is proven to be medically essential for good health. What's a rational person or doctor to do? The answer: test to ensure sufficient iron without jeopardizing safety.

It was Nutri-Chem's approach of investigating simplistic arguments and contradictory statements that led to the funding by the National Research Council of Canada of our ICMT laboratory. Our purpose is to investigate a complete range of nutritional parameters in Down Syndrome. Distinguished scientists such as Dr. Keith Ingold[1] from the Research Council

## WHAT WILL I LEARN?

▸ How MSB could benefit your child.

▸ The role of testing in determining what's right for your child.

▸ How common dietary deficiencies could sabotage your child's health.

▸ How Metalife Biomedical Center's integrated medical approach could help you and your child.

*of Canada had extensive experience with vitamin E. They were aware that it is one of the few therapies proven effective in treatment of Alzheimer's disease. I brought to their attention the fact that virtually all individuals with Down Syndrome develop Alzheimer's. There was mutual agreement that in light of this fact, it is remarkable that testing is not routinely done for the prevention or treatment of Alzheimer's in Down Syndrome. Research Council scientists saw the logic in establishing optimal ranges for vitamin E for this purpose.*

*Biochemically speaking, it was a natural progression to go on to measure all elements of nutrition and their impact on health (the core purpose of our ICMT lab). vitamin E is but one leg of many that support optimal health, a view not shared by traditional pharmacists who subscribe to a single-treatment approach. When I think like such a pharmacist, I lose sight of how insufficient one leg is in supporting the table of health. When I think as a biochemist, I recognize that health needs the support of many legs in the form of proper balance of nutrients. – K.M.*

## MSB – A nutritional supplement designed for children with Down Syndrome

Parents demanding the best for their children – this is the real story behind many of the advancements on behalf of children with Down Syndrome. And it's the story behind the development of Nutri-Chem's MSB formula.

Almost 20 years ago, well before the technical advancement of the ICMT clinical laboratory, I met with a group of parents of children with Down Syndrome. They asked me to review work done by Dr. Henry Turkel on vitamin therapies for children with Down Syndrome. From my perspective as a pharmacist trained in biochemistry and specializing in nutritional supplements, I analyzed Turkel's research. I then met with the parents and made recommendations on how such a nutritional formula could be improved to benefit their children with Down Syndrome. And the parents demanded that I do just that.

During the early phase of my involvement with Down Syndrome, I did something that seemed logical to me but proved rare in medical circles. I read all the literature. It was only later that I realized how such a basic form of education is uncommon.

In collaboration with Nutri-Chem staff, researchers, doctors and the parents themselves, the first MSB formula was developed. It combines vitamins, minerals, amino acids and enzymes with a special emphasis on antioxidants to enhance your child's immune system. The supplement is specifically formulated to supply nutrients proven to be inadequate in children with Down Syndrome, as well as to supply the most metabolically active form of nutrients. Nutri-Chem uses safe ingredients of the highest quality in compounding MSB.

Since 1983, when Nutri-Chem introduced its MSB nutritional supplement for children with Down Syndrome, the formula has undergone several updates. These changes have reflected new scientific evidence, and the results shown in laboratory tests of children who use MSB. The most recent version, MSBPlus V6, represents a breakthrough in taste in response to complaints by parents and their children. In their natural state, vitamins, minerals and amino acids do not have a pleasant taste. Most commercial supplements use a sugar to make them palatable, but parents told Nutri-Chem they wanted to keep MSB sugar-free. The solution, "Southern Splash," a flavouring, passed the children's taste test and met the requirements of parents. Since not all MSB clients use version 6, Southern Splash can be added to all previous formulas. MSB supplements are available in powder form with Southern Splash which is mixed with liquid and drunk as a beverage, and in capsule form for older children.

Your child should take MSB with food and, if possible, spread throughout the day with meals. Dosage will depend on your child's age and weight.

# Supplement Facts

Serving Size
Servings Per Container

| Amount Per Serving | % Daily Value for Children Under 4 Years of Age | % Daily Value for Adults* and Children 4 or more Years of Age | Amount Per Serving | % Daily Value for Children Under 4 Years of Age | % Daily Value for Adults* and Children 4 or more Years of Age |
|---|---|---|---|---|---|
| Vitamin A | | | L-Methionine | | |
| Beta-carotene | | | L-Cysteine | | |
| Vitamin C | | | L-Ornithine | | |
| Vitamin D | | | L-Lysine | | |
| Vitamin E | | | L-Taurine | | |
| B1 | | | L-Proline | | |
| B2 | | | L-Serine | | |
| B3 | | | L-Tyrosine | | |
| Vitamin B6 | | | L-Phenylalanine | | |
| Folic Acid | | | Alpha-ketoglutaric acid | | |
| Vitamin B12 | | | Acetyl-l-carnitine | | |
| Biotin | | | Lipoic Acid | | |
| B5 | | | Pancreatic Enzymes | | |
| Calcium | | | Betaine HCL | | |
| Iron | | | Inositol | | |
| Iodine | | | Bromelain | | |
| Magnesium | | | Papain | | |
| Zinc | | | Choline Dihydrogen Citrate | | |
| Selenium | | | DMAE | | |
| Manganese | | | Glutathion | | |
| Chromium | | | Coenzyme Q10 | | |
| Molybdenum | | | The MacLeod Mix | | |
| Potassium | | | (Phosphatidyl-serine, Lycopenes, | | |
| Bioflavonoids | | | Grape Seed extract, | | |
| | | | Mixed Carotenoids, Folinic acid, | | |
| | | | Methylcobalamin, | | |
| | | | Natural fruit flavoring) | | |

* Percent Daily Values are based on a 2,000 calorie diet

† Daily Value not established

# MSB side effects

Nutri-Chem has 20 years worth of recorded data on side effects from thousands of MSB users. While this reporting system is a voluntary one, it replicates the identical system to report adverse reactions in any medication. By far the most common reported adverse reaction is gastrointestinal-related with loose stool being the most frequent. This effect appears to be dose-related as decreasing dosage seems to improve the problem in most cases.

Other adverse reactions reported include:

- skin reactions (rashes or reddening);
- central nervous system effects (sleeplessness and agitation the most common – improvement of this effect seems related to folate cycle disturbances);
- yellowing of skin (two reported cases, both of which improved with zinc supplementation).

Overall the reported rate of adverse effects from supplementation is less than one percent (1%). This number is actually less than the number of reports we would receive from a placebo. This means that we have fewer reported side effects than if we were giving sugar tablets. Of course, we understand that everybody doesn't report every side effect with a vitamin. However, it does give us assurance as to safety. There has never been a reported death with the use of any supplements in the U.S.A. or Canada in the range Nutri-Chem is using them. (Compare this to the 100,000 deaths per year in U.S. hospitals from drug use alone.[2])

# Testing and individualization

Asking why you should have laboratory testing done on your child is like asking why you get your oil checked on your car. Why not just drive your car around until it runs out of oil and stops? The answer is pretty obvious: you can prevent problems and keep things in good working order by checking your car's oil level and replenishing it when it's low.

Unlike school tests, there is no pass or fail grade in metabolic testing. The goal is prevention and remediation – to stop problems before they happen, and to fix problems once they've occurred.

Testing not only allows you to determine specific nutrient levels, it can also give you a picture of what's happening in your child's body if the results are analyzed by a knowledgeable nutritional biochemist.

## Zinc testing

Testing for nutritional deficiencies is inherently controversial. If we look at zinc and folic acid, we can see why. Physicians have successfully argued (and with good reason) that testing for harmful folic acid deficiency adds unnecessary cost. Instead, they argue, why not just administer folic acid regardless of testing because of its known safety and benefit in preventing neuro tube defects. Why, then do doctors insist that where Down Syndrome is concerned any zinc supplementation must be preceded by testing? This attitude is also seen with regard to zinc supplementation despite its recommendation by the Medical Advisory Board of the National Down Syndrome Congress.[3]

In my 20 years of work with Down Syndrome, I have rarely encountered a physician who tests for zinc levels. I'd like to think this anti-testing bias might be support in disguise – maybe doctors actually believe that zinc should be routinely administered for its efficacy and safety much like folic acid. Or maybe they recognize that, like folic acid, testing blood levels is actually a poor indicator of zinc levels. Unfortunately, experience teaches me none of this is the case. Physician resistance is rooted in bias against nutritional therapies in Down Syndrome because of the condition's genetic component.

Parents should have their children tested for plasma zinc as recommended by Dr. S. Pueschel.[4] Plasma zinc levels should be at least 100 micrograms per dl (ug/dl), the average for non-Down Syndrome controls. Blood levels may not accurately reflect actual tissue levels of zinc. In addition, parents should note that zinc levels in non-Down Syndrome control groups are commonly deficient. Taken together, these facts complicate the picture for zinc testing. Because of zinc's proven ability to improve thyroid and immune function and affect growth, testing is important. However, parents should consider supplementation regardless of testing, particularly until a reliable testing method is available.

Two tests are under investigation to measure the activity of a zinc-dependent hormone. One such test involves plasma thymic hormone (STF), the hormone that stimulates T-lymphoctye blood cells that attack invading organisms. These cells are proven low in Down Syndrome and extremely responsive to zinc supplementation.[5] The other test is for hepatic 5 D-1 which again is highly responsive to zinc supplementation and affects conversion of T4 to T3. In other words, a more sensitive indicator of zinc levels would be an impaired immune system and low thyroid which is what we commonly find in Down Syndrome anyway!

## T3 and T4

The common thyroid medications eltroxin and synthroid are actually brand names for T4. These medications require the zinc-dependent enzyme 5D-1 to convert this T4 to the biologically active T3. This is why individuals with Down Syndrome should use a T3-containing product along with zinc if they require thyroid therapy. A complete thyroid such as amour thyroid which contains T3 improved cognitive function significantly better than a simple T4 supplement.[6]

# Iron testing

Iron testing is universally available and gives an accurate reflection of what is going on in the body. There's no controversy about the essential need for iron for growth, development, a healthy immune system and other functions.

Yet many parents have been told that iron is harmful for their children with Down Syndrome. Children with Down Syndrome should have a routine CBC (complete blood count) which includes hemoglobin and hematocrit. It also gives the size and hemoglobin concentration of the red blood cells which are early warning signs of anemias, potential B-vitamin deficiencies like folic acid and $B_{12}$ and other more serious disorders. Ferritin is the protein with which iron is stored and is a first very sensitive indicator of iron deficiency.

What parents often don't realize is that it's not necessary to use more and more iron to improve iron stores. In fact, iron absorption can be improved by as much as 10 times by the type of iron, the presence of acid and the type of protein that it is consumed with. Nutri-Chem uses an iron citrate chelate along with ascorbic acid to enhance absorption. If further indicated, the use of a whey protein with lacto ferrin instead of casein protein will improve iron absorption by as much as five times. This knowledge is used in the infant formula industry. The fact is that iron deficiency is a relatively common problem which can be addressed in a safe, effective fashion.

The CBC test detects abnormalities of blood cells where they tend to get bigger and fatter. This can be related to a deficiency of folic acid, iron and $B_{12}$. In fact, iron deficiency can mask the symptoms of folic acid and $B_{12}$ deficiencies. Any increase in size in red blood cells requires additional testing of $B_{12}$, folic acid and iron to find out why. There are a variety of more sophisticated and functional tests to determine the cause of these irregularities. For example, folic acid and folinic acid testing, free iron and iron binding capacity, ferritin as previously noted, vitamin $B_{12}$ and methyl melonic acid may be used. These tests should be done on your child's regular check up.

Nutri-Chem also recommends:

- **SCREENING TESTS FOR CELIAC DISEASE** are recommended by the Medical Advisory Committee of the Down Syndrome

Congress. These should be done on all children regardless of whether or not they have symptoms.

- **THYROID (TSH) TESTING.** A complete thyroid panel including TSH and free T3 and free T4.

- **ZINC AND COPPER TESTING.** Remember results may poorly reflect tissue levels but testing must still be done.

- **OXYMARK PROFILE.** The oxymark profile comprises of four categories of testing. See sidebar for details.

Analysis of the laboratory test results is complex. It involves not just identifying a deficiency, but why a deficiency or abnormality exists. Nutrients are not like drugs – they do not act in isolation, so it is vital that not only a deficiency or excess be identified, but also that its impact on other biochemical pathways be considered.

Testing allows your child's nutritional supplement to be individualized and tailored to her or his specific needs. Individualized compounds not only correct nutritional conditions, they can remove substances to which your child is

## Oxymark profile

This profile comprises four categories of testing:

**1. Antioxidant levels and oxidative stress.** Vitamin E and coenzyme Q10 levels should be in the upper range of normal, and vitamin A levels above average. Alpha carotene reflects fruit and vegetable consumption and should encompass food guide requirements of five or more servings daily (most kids don't come close!).

**2. Amino acids.** Testing may reflect protein malnutrition, deficiency or excess of methylation intermediates, deficiency of precursors for seratonin and dopamine and metabolic abnormalities.

**3. Urinary organic acids.** They indicate deficiencies of B12, B vitamins, glutathione, magnesium, carnitine, co enzyme Q10 and other essential nutrients. Toxic elements such as heavy metals and parasites and toxic chemicals can also be indicated through urinary organic acid testing.

**4. Red blood cell fatty acids.** The red blood cell membrane is an accurate reflection of brain composition. Certain key essential fatty acids have been proven to affect mood. These are significantly altered in schizophrenia, attention focus disorders and Alzheimer's disease. Measurement of these elements encourages restriction of saturated fats and fried foods in the diet. It encourages the use of healthy essential oils from fish and vegetables. Specific supplemental oils can be used when necessary.

allergic, strengthen dosage of specific ingredients or remove ingredients that cause a negative reaction when taken in combination with other medications your child is on.

## How to read blood tests

**A Complete Blood Count, known as a CBC,** is a routine test that should be done on your child at regular intervals, together with an iron panel.

The CBC measures the cellular (or formed) elements of blood, and calculates a "value" for each. There is a normal range associated with these values, and any deviation should be discussed thoroughly with your child's physician.

The CBC is a useful test for the determination of everything from simple conditions such as anemia, to more complex problems such as hypothyroidism. Elevated MCV levels may indicate disturbances in DNA synthesis, and can be an early warning symptom for leukemia.

The values commonly included in a CBC test include:

- **white blood cell count (CBC)**, referred to as the leukocyte count: the number of white blood cells in a volume of blood;

- **white cell differential**: the percentage of different types of white blood cells;

- **red cell count (RBC)**: the number of red blood cells in a volume of blood;

- **hemoglobin (Hb)**: the amount of hemoglobin (protein molecule that carries oxygen and gives blood its red colour) in a volume of blood;

- **hematocrit (Hct)**: the ratio of the volume of red cells to the volume of whole blood (differs between sexes);

- **mean cell volume (MCV)**: the average volume of a red cell;

- **mean cell hemoglobin (MCH)**: the average amount of hemoglobin in the average red cell;

- **mean cell hemoglobin concentration (MCHC)**: the average concentration of hemoglobin in a given volume of red cells;

- **red cell distribution width (RDW)**: measurement of the variability of red cell size;

- **platelet count**: the number of platelets (fragments of cytoplasm from a cell found in the bone marrow) found in a volume of blood.

# Completing the picture

Correcting nutritional deficiencies and metabolic disturbances with vitamin supplements is only one half of the picture. Metabolic testing will also indicate what changes are needed in your child's diet. Taken together, a healthy diet and appropriate supplements give your child complete nutritional support for both mind and body.

---

# Closing comments from Kent:

*In 20 years of talking with Nutri-Chem clients about their diets, I've never yet met a person who says their doctor ever actually asked them what they're eating. This is the basic starting point for giving nutritional advice about diets. When I speak to our clients, I don't ask "What do you eat for breakfast, lunch and dinner?" I ask them "What did you eat yesterday?". It's this focus on the individual and what they're actually consuming that gets to the root of the problem. It's not magic. Most people, when they're faced with the increasing problem of obesity in children, take the absolute wrong approach. They deny their child food. This only creates nutritional starvation and worsens the problem by reducing lean muscle mass. Instead, they should adjust their child's diet so that the child consumes the right balance of protein and amino acids throughout the day, while reducing the amount of carbohydrates in the diet and decreasing the bad fats while increasing consumption of fish or fish oil supplements.*

*I am often asked by parents whether or not they should have testing done on their son or daughter. Following are the three issues you should consider as a parent in answering this question.*

1. *Cost. Additional testing not typically covered by insurance is approximately $500 U.S. or $750 Cdn. By additional, I mean tests that aren't considered "routine." Ideally all individuals with Down Syndrome should be tested annually because even one nutrient deficiency can be devastating. This speaks to the prevention versus treatment issue. Most of the medical system is geared toward treatment. The question you need to answer for yourself is should you wait for symptoms to appear or find out about a problem before things reach that stage. If testing is not affordable for your family, then I suggest using our basic nutritional supplement formula for Down Syndrome. It will offer your child a complete compound covering the nutrients we know are required in Down Syndrome. Even when a child is basically well, we find that we can bring nutrients up to an optimal range that counteracts deficiencies in diet due to our hurried, hectic modern lifestyles.*

*If a problem remains unresolved, lab testing becomes important. For another perspective on the cost issue, consider that one routine ear infection is estimated to cost the average family in the order of $1,100 (U.S.) from lost work time, drugs, etc.*

## A new approach to medical treatment

Many of my clients come to me because they are frustrated and discouraged about how their children's health issues are being managed. Often, the medical approach does not marry into the fundamentals of nutrition, metabolism and hormones. In an effort to provide much-needed medical support to these clients, and to address the problem of a non-integrated approach to their health, I recently created the Metalife Biomedical Center in Ottawa, Canada. At the Metalife Biomedical Center, we have integrated medical doctors, nurses, registered nutritional consultants, naturopaths, biochemists and pharmacists under my direction, to create a medical center where fundamental nutrition, biochemical and hormonal issues are medically managed by our team of experts.

2. *Inconvenience. Drawing blood from your child, shipping tests via courier, and other tasks may seem too much for a busy doctor to consider. That's why parents need to consider this step themselves.*

3. *Controversy. Strange as this may seem, much of this controversy stems from taking an integrative approach to testing when the individual tests themselves make undisputed sense. Because of medical scepticism, many parents don't tell their child's medical doctor they are taking vitamin therapies for fear of recrimination. Our approach at Nutri-Chem is to encourage dialogue between patients and their doctors. Many physicians come to appreciate the science of using clinical laboratory testing to assess nutrients. – K.M.*

---

In our medical center, we treat children and adults from around the world. Our approach is straightforward: while other medical centers often rely on too narrow a spectrum of healthcare professionals and treatments, we seek input from a wide range of professionals and explore many potential treatments. At Metalife Biomedical, our doctors and other professionals are constantly pushing the envelope to find the best complementary and conventional medical treatments for our clients, both adults and children.

For more information on our approach, contact us directly at:
Metalife Biomedical Center
Telephone: (613) 721-3669
Fax: (613) 829-2226
E-mail: info@metalifebiomedical.com
Website: www.metalifebiomedical.com

# Endnotes

1. Dr. Keith Ingold has co-authored over 150 research papers. A sample: Vitamin E for coronary bypass operations. A prospective, double-blind, randomized trial. Journal of Thoracic and Cardiovascular Surgery. 1994 Aug;108(2):302-310.

   "Application of deuterated alpha-tocopherols to the biokinetics and bioavailability of vitamin E." *Free Radical Research Communications.* 1990;11(1-3):99-107.

   "Vitamin E as an in vitro and in vivo antioxidant." *Annals of the New York Academy of Science.* 1989;570:7-22.

   "The relative contributions of vitamin E, urate, ascorbate and proteins to the total peroxyl radical-trapping antioxidant activity of human blood plasma." *Biochimica Biophysica Acta.* 1987 Jun 22;924(3):408-419.

   "First proof that vitamin E is major lipid-soluble, chain-breaking antioxidant in human blood plasma." *Lancet.* 1982 Aug 7;2 (8293): 327

2. Barbara Starfield, (2000) "Is US Health Really the Best in the World?" *Journal of the American Medical Association*, 284: 483-5

3. Pueschel, S. (1999) "Gastrointestinal concerns and nutritional issues in persons with Down syndrome." *Down Syndrome Quarterly* 4(4): 1-11.

4. Pueschel, S. (1999) "Gastrointestinal concerns and nutritional issues in persons with Down syndrome." *Down Syndrome Quarterly* 4(4): 1-11.

5. Franceschi, C. et al. (1988) "Oral zinc supplementation in Down's syndrome: restoration of thymic endocrine activity and of some immune defects." *Journal of Mental Deficiency Research* 32: 169-181.

6. Banevicius, R., et al (1999) "Effects of thyroxine as compared with thyroxine plus triiodothyronine in patients with hypothyroidism." *New England Journal of Medicine* 1999 Feb. 11; 340(6): 469-70

# CHAPTER 14

# RESEARCH FOR TOMORROW

---

*HAVE YOU EVER SPENT HOURS TEARING THE HOUSE APART WHILE YOU LOOK for some missing item, only to find that it was right under your nose all along? If so, you understand the frustration of nutritional scientists who face a medical community that says "we have to keep looking" for answers we already have. – K.M.*

---

## When is enough research enough?

We have research proving this antioxidant vitamin slows the progression of Alzheimer's disease in moderate cases,[1] and has probable benefits for the heart.[2, 3, 4, 5, 6] We have research using antioxidant vitamin E on the brains of Down Syndrome fetuses that found it stabilized and regenerated brain cells causing the cells to grow and thrive until they looked like normal cells.[7] And we have research on seniors using vitamin E plus a multiple vitamin that dramatically reduced their number of sick days.[8, 9, 10] Do we have enough research into the benefits of vitamin E? The answer is yes, and no. Yes, we have enough research to support using

> **WHAT WILL I LEARN?**
>
> - What answers do we already have about the usefulness of nutritional therapies?
>
> - Should we wait for conclusive proof?
>
> - What answers do we still need to search for?

vitamin E now without the need to "keep on looking." We know it's beneficial and safe. No, we don't have enough research if we want to go one step further: to conclusively prove the plausible theory that it prevents diseases. This will need long-term studies of several decades' duration, so the definitive answer on prevention can't be known for some time.

Where children with Down Syndrome are concerned, critics of vitamin therapy continue to refute any benefits because research has not been conducted on this particular group of children. Again using vitamin E as an example, existing research on populations who do not have Down Syndrome but who share the same problems of neurological deterioration, prove that vitamin E slows brain cell death. Yet vitamin critics find the use of drugs preferable despite the potential for harmful side effects presented by some drugs.

As we've seen in the chapter on studies, research exists within an environment that includes biases (of researchers and of subjects), methodological flaws, subjective interpretations and corporate interests where huge profits are at stake. These factors don't diminish the need for research, but they should provide us with some perspective to question the five w's of medical research: who's behind it, what was studied, when did the study take place, where was it conducted and why was the study carried out?

## The road ahead

If I could have a wish list for research, top on my list would be an investigation into how far nutritional therapies can go in terms of preventing or reversing disease. We have sufficient research to be able to claim that vitamins (in supplements and in the food we eat) can promote health at recommended levels of safety. What we need, and what I would love to know as a nutritional biochemist, is what the upper optimal limits are for specific nutrients. Could we reverse or fix certain conditions with higher doses or combinations of nutrients?

As far as Down Syndrome is concerned, we need further study on the potential for antioxidant vitamins such as vitamin E. How much can we improve the immune system and eliminate brain cell degeneration? We need to know more about folate metabolism and metabolic disturbances in the SAM cycle. Can we normalize this metabolic pathway with sufficient quantities of the right nutrients to prevent the onset of leukemia? What metabolic disturbances in mothers pose risk factors? What are the links between Down Syndrome, leukemia and Autism? In terms of I.Q., we already know that brain function can be improved with diet and supplements. How far could dietary methods and supplements be used to prevent low I.Q.?

The human genome project has drawn a great deal of attention and scientific research. It is mapping the human genetic code that determines everything about us. Scientists predict that once the mapping is complete (and understood), we will be able to diagnose what diseases a person will get, and then manipulate genes or design drugs tailored to that person's individual genetic makeup. This holds the promise that disease will be eradicated and genetic birth defects eliminated. Yet any benefits from this research are many years (and many billions of dollars of research money) away. In the meantime, we haven't explored the potential for safe, natural substances – food and vitamins – that are right under our noses.

What gene mapping has done is show that if you improve the physical expression of a gene there is actual feedback to modify the genetic expression. What this means is if you have a genetic expression of a small arm, and you use exercise and nutrients to maximize the size of the arm, then its genetic code is altered. This leads us to wonder whether we could affect the genetic code for Down Syndrome through such nutritional interventions as zinc supplementation. Typically we have been taught that genetic modifications are possible only through high-tech, costly gene manipulation. Ultimately the best way to alter our genetic structure just may be by living well, exercising and supplying our body with missing or incomplete nutrients and materials.

In the end, when we talk about health colliding with the environment, nutrients and genetics, we just may find that genetics play a very minor role in this triangle. In our high-technology medical world, we can define what it is to be sick. But we have no idea what it is we need to be healthy beyond simple platitudes telling us to eat a balanced diet and exercise. The fundamental first step is to optimize our range of nutrients.

Do you know what an optimal diet consists of? Have you had your child's metabolic testing done? Is your child anemic? How is your child's bowel functioning? What are your child's zinc levels? While we're researching how to change the world, have we looked at what's right under our noses?

# Endnotes

1. Sano, M., et al. (1997) "A controlled trial of selegiline, alpha-tocopherol, or both as treatment for Alzheimer's disease." *New England Journal of Medicine* 336: 1216-22.

2. Losonczy, K., et al. (1996) "Vitamin E and C supplement use and risk of all-cause and coronary heart disease mortality in older persons: the Established Populations for Epidemiologic Studies of the Elderly." *American Journal of Clinical Nutrition* 64: 190-6

3. Stephens, N.B., et al. (1996) "Randomised controlled trial of vitamin E in patients with coronary disease: Cambridge Heart Antioxidant Study (CHAOS)." *Lancet* 347: 781-86.

4. Rimm, E., et al. (1993) "Vitamin E consumption and the risk of coronary heart disease in men." *New England Journal of Medicine* 328: 1450-6.

5. Stampfer, M., et al. (1993) "Vitamin E consumption and the risk of coronary disease in women." *New England Journal of Medicine* 328: 1450-6

6. Yusuf, S., et al. (2000) *Vitamin E supplementation and cardiovascular events in high-risk patients. The Heart Outcomes Prevention Evaluation Study Investigators.* 342: 154-60.

7. Busciglio, J., and Yanker, B.A. (1995) "Apoptosis and increased generation of reactive oxygen species in Down's syndrome neurons in vitro." *Nature* 378: 776-79.

8. Meydani, S., et al. (1997) "Vitamin E supplementation and in vivo immune response in healthy elderly subjects." *Journal of the American Medical Association* 277: 1380-86.

9. Chandra, R (1992) "Effect of vitamin and trace-element supplementation on immune responses and infection in elderly subjects." *Lancet* 340: 1124-27.

10. Pike, J., and Chandra, R.K. (1995) "Effect of vitamin and trace element supplementation on immune indices in healthy elderly." *International Journal of Vitamin and Nutrition Research* 65: 117-20.

# APPENDICES

## APPENDIX A
### EXISTING STUDIES AND THEIR LIMITATIONS

## APPENDIX B
### GLOSSARY

# EXISTING STUDIES AND THEIR LIMITATIONS

*I spoke about nutrition in Down Syndrome at a conference at the National Down Syndrome Congress in Phoenix, Arizona a few years ago. It was actually my first head-to-head experience with the absolute and vicious attack on the use of nutritional supplements in Down Syndrome. That attack came from Dr. S. M. Pueschel. Part of the animosity directed at me was based on the fact that I was making money on nutritional supplements. From my perspective this is ridiculous because of existing evidence that for many health issues related to Down Syndrome, nutrients are safe and effective while drugs have proven ineffective with significant risks. As a pharmacist my income is derived from the sale of drugs, vitamins and other remedies. Some are of benefit, some are not. Medical doctors derive their income from the prescription of treatments, some of which will be of benefit, and some not.*

## WHAT WILL I LEARN?

▸ Why you need to know who funds medical studies.

▸ How study bias could affect your child's health options.

▸ The problems with one important anti-vitamin study.

*No professional (including doctors) can or should disassociate their practise from the economic benefits it provides. What puzzles and irritates me is the pretense that drug therapies are promoted for their health benefits devoid of any economic interests, while vitamins and nutritional therapy are characterized as motivated by profit alone. To put some perspective on this situation, it is useful to note that in a New England Journal of Medicine reported study, not one medical doctor could be found who did not have a direct or indirect financial interest in a pharmaceutical company.*[1] – *K.M.*

## Who pays the piper?

In 1999, the *Journal of the American Medical Association* (JAMA) reported on a study finding that "pharmaceutical company-sponsored studies were less likely than nonprofit-sponsored studies to report unfavorable qualitative conclusions."[2] Translation: companies who pay for results don't like to report on bad results. This is one of many recent articles and reports concerned with scientific objectivity and bias. "Is Academic Medicine for Sale?" asked a *New England Journal of Medicine* article in May, 2000.[3] In another case, doctors offered opinions on both sides of a sensitive topic in response to a *JAMA* article,"Physicians and the pharmaceutical industry: is a gift ever just a gift?"[4]

Understandably, dedicated researchers and physicians feel a certain defensiveness when their commitment to scientific inquiry and patient health is questioned. Doctors deny that drug companies tell them when and what to prescribe to their patients. Others acknowledge the effect company gifts and marketing have on physician behaviour and worry about the increasing corporate sponsorship of professional journals and education conferences. Why do they worry? Where research is concerned, the pharmaceutical industry is a primary source of financial support and study publication.

## Searching out bias

Bias is a complex issue. It can be subtle and unconscious. However, with health, indeed life itself, at stake, it is important to dig beneath the surface and recognize the context in which research studies are conducted.

The first place that bias can become an issue in research studies is in the hypothesis itself. What you set out to find will determine the parameters of your results. The frame of reference of the researcher is critical – what attitude, school of thought, experience, does the researcher bring to the study? Is the researcher looking to prove that something is beneficial, or to prove that it is not? Does the researcher want to measure only dramatic outcomes at the expense of more subtle, yet significant, results?

When a study is funded by industry the design of the study is set up to maximize potentially observed benefits of the drug. This makes sense if you are paying for the study because you want your drug to get a positive trial. Invariably when supplements have been studied in Down Syndrome, the potential benefits are ignored because there is no inherent vested interest in showing that vitamins are beneficial.

## What's the study's 'power'?

Next to hypothesis, the study's methodology is crucial. How are the study's subjects chosen? Who is included, and who excluded, from participation? How many will be studied, and for how long? These last two (number studied and length of time) comprise what is known as the "power" of the study. This is of particular importance when a study purports to measure the effects of an intervention on something as complex as intelligence. Such a study will need a high power to show any meaningful results. Yet nutritional benefits for children with Down Syndrome are regularly disputed on the basis of studies lacking sufficient power. These studies have been designed to fail, with timeframes as low as one month. These same studies also illustrate the principle that "a study only proves what it set out to prove," concentrating as they have on I.Q., with little regard for other significant improvements such as greater alertness and fewer infections which may lead to intellectual improvements over time.

The type of study can influence outcome also. Typically, observational studies are discounted as unscientific, yet they often indicate important improvements that would otherwise be ignored. Randomized, controlled trials are considered the "gold standard" of evaluation for the efficacy of a treatment. The truth is that there is no perfect method, and randomized, controlled studies have limitations of their own. These include some of the factors mentioned above (size and length of study), as well as a failure to address long-term consequences, both positive and negative. There are far too many cases where studies have proven efficacy and safety of a treatment that is later found to be unsafe and withdrawn from use, often after tragedies have occurred.

As well as the attitude and bias of the researcher, the participants themselves – and in the case of children, their parents and caregivers – bring with them a set of attitudes and behaviours. It is virtually impossible to control for all variables that may influence outcomes.

## A case in point

When we look at the limitations of existing studies on nutrition and children with Down Syndrome, the first problem we encounter is just how few such studies exist. How is it that there is so little scientific interest in studying the benefits of nutritional therapies for children with Down Syndrome, when there is widespread medical condemnation of the efficacy of vitamins for this population?

One study often cited as proof that vitamin A is of no benefit for children with Down Syndrome was conducted in 1990 by Dr. S. M. Pueschel, et al, entitled "Vitamin A gastrointestinal absorption in persons with Down's (sic) Syndrome."[5] Because of the negative impact this study has had, it is useful to examine its methodology and results. A study summary follows, with observations about its limitations:

- The study set out to determine whether or not vitamin A absorption was a problem in children with Down Syndrome. It cited "flaws in study design" of earlier studies that had had conflicting results.

- The study included 33 patients with Down Syndrome and 14 intellectually normal persons (control group) for comparison. Dietary histories were conducted to determine that both groups' daily intake met the recommended daily allowance of vitamin A, and that there was no significant difference in vitamin A intake between the two groups.

- Vitamin A absorption was measured at 0, 3, and 6-hour intervals.

- The study found that the vitamin A absorption in the persons with Down Syndrome paralleled that of the normal individuals and that there was no significant difference of vitamin A levels between study and comparison groups except for the 6-hour values. It concluded that "these investigations do not support previous reports of significantly decreased vitamin A absorption in individuals with Down's Syndrome."

There are three main problems with Dr. Pueschel's study. These relate to the study group selected, the form of vitamin A administered, and the conclusions reached by the investigators.

First, the study group of persons with Down Syndrome did NOT include anyone with the following: low protein intake, decreased zinc levels, thyroid disorders and infections – all of which occur with high frequency in people with Down Syndrome and were acknowledged by the researchers to be possible causes of interference with vitamin A. Therefore, the study excluded the very population with Down Syndrome most likely to have vitamin A disturbances and to benefit from supplements.

Second, the form of vitamin A used was water-soluble. There is no such form found in the diet. Naturally-occurring vitamin A is fat-soluble, and by using a water-soluble synthetic form, absorption was altered and greatly enhanced.

Finally, the conclusion of this study is not supported by its findings. Dr. Pueschel's study group exhibited "significantly reduced vitamin A levels in the Down's Syndrome group at 6 hours following vitamin A administration." This is indicative of vitamin A disturbances in one of several important areas: absorption, distribution, metabolism or excretion. By choosing to look only at absorption, and by ignoring the findings at hour 6, the conclusion was reached that no difference existed between the Down Syndrome and control groups.

In fact, the study could have been read to support vitamin A disturbances based on its findings. It could have indicated that, even though the highest-absorbing form of vitamin A was used, and despite the fact that no people with interfering conditions common in Down Syndrome were included, there were significantly lower levels of vitamin A after 6 hours.

Dr. Pueschel's study is considered THE definitive proof against vitamin A deficiencies in people with Down Syndrome. If you view this study as flawed in its design and outcome, the question arises as to why it should be used to inhibit nutritional supplements for children with Down Syndrome.

The bias of the medical community is illustrated in a recent statement made by Dr. Pueschel in a statement entitled "Gastrointestinal Concerns and Nutritional Issues In Persons with Down Syndrome"[6] where in the beginning summary it states "there is ample evidence that supplemental vitamins and minerals do not benefit the child's cognitive and physical abilities. There are, however certain trace elements and minerals such as selenium and zinc as well as specific antioxidants that may be deficient and need to be administered to the child with Down Syndrome. A number of diseases such as congenital heart disease, thyroid disorders and celiac disease can interfere with adequate nutrition and these children often need nutritional assistance." This statement by Dr. Pueschel is tantamount to me concluding that drugs are all bad for you – unless of course you need drugs, and then you would need to take them because you are in fact someone that needs them!

## Other important studies

In a study by Lucas et al, reported in the British Medical Journal in 1998, researchers examined the effects of vitamin supplementation on the developing brains of premature babies.[7]

This study had over 483 participants all age matched and in similar socio-economic conditions. The participants were premature babies who are at significant risks for mental delay. In the study, half the children, at a very young age (less than 2 years old) were given for one month ONLY an enriched nutrient formula. The other children received placebos. Although enriched, the formula was not mega-vitamin therapy of the type used in the early 1980s by Dr. R. Harrell (whose study we will look at later in this section). After a minimum of 5 years, at the average age of 7, the I.Q. of all these children was assessed. It is important to take note that the authors of the study wrote that it was crucial to give nutrients at an age of 2 years or less when the brain was developing, but at they same time they could only assess the I.Q. of these children when they reached the age of 7. It was only at this time that they could get an accurate I.Q. measurement. The results of this study were that there was a significant and dramatic improvement in I.Q. in the supplemented group of children taking the enriched formula.

Unfortunately, the studies involving children with Down Syndrome are not as clear, in my opinion, because they are not as well designed and well followed up as, for instance, this British study was. For example, in the studies involving children with Down Syndrome, we have low numbers of subjects (ranging from as few as 4 subjects to as many as 56). We have short terms of investigation (ranging from 4 to 8 months). We have mega doses of vitamins being used versus doses approximating the RDA. We have no studies of nutrition in children younger than 2 years of age (critical if we're interested in the impact of supplementation on brain development). In fact, what is most striking about this British premature children study is that the supplements were given for a period of only one month and the timing of what stage in a child's life they were given was noted to be important.

What do the studies have to say? Following is a summary of some of the important ones.

1. **WEATHERS ET AL**[8]

   Number of subjects:  47

   Ages: 6 to 17 years

   Subject given: Megavitamins according to formula of Dr. Harrell, 4 month duration

   Study design: Placebo given, not blinded, matching of subjects

   Result: No significant difference in I.Q.

   Other commentary: Parents whose children were on supplements chose to continue on supplements even though the study held that there was no benefit.

2. **HARRELL ET AL**[9]

   Number of subjects: 4

   Ages: 5-9 years

   Subject given: Harrell's formula and thyroid supplement, 4 months of supplement then 4 months of placebo OR 4 months of placebo then 4 months of supplement

   Study design: Small numbers, matching, assessor was not "blinded"

   Result: Significant improvement in I.Q. on supplements

   Other commentary: This is the one positive study that attracted much attention to recreate its results. Too small a number of subjects to prove.

3. **COBURN ET AL**[10]

Number of subjects: 4

Ages: 21-29 years

Subject given: Megavitamins according to Dr. Harrell's formulation, 5 months duration

Study design: small number, institutionalized

Result: No significant benefit to I.Q. for subjects on supplements

Other commentary: Insufficient numbers and duration to prove anything

4. **SMITH ET AL**[11]

Number of subjects: 56

Ages: 7-15 years

Subject given: Megavitamin formula according to Dr. Harrell, 8 months duration (4 on supplement, 4 off)

Study design: Matched by cognitive level, age, sex, socio-economic status

Result: No significant benefit to I.Q.

Other commentary: There WERE in fact significant effects. Using the Weshcler Intelligence Scale, they did find a significance difference in intelligence scales for children on supplements. Furthermore 8 out of 12 subtests showed significant benefits but were ignored in an unexplained fashion. For the group treated with supplements: "For 8 of sub-test comparisons (of 9) there were significant time main effects but because they did not bear on the major question of study so they were not reported." In the supplement group, 2 of 5 had significant improvement while in the placebo group all had decrease in I.Q.

This study was among the best-designed of this group, and Smith et al actually found significant improvements. But they chose not report these improvements because "it did not impact on the objective of the study." The object of the study was to disprove Dr. Harrell's hypothesis.

## 5. BENNETT ET AL[12]

Number of subjects: 20 children

Ages: 5 to 13; all functioned at less than kindergarten level

Subjects given: Megavitamins according to Dr. Harrell's formula, 8 month duration

Study design: Double blinded

Result: No significant benefits

Other commentary: It is interesting to note that by age five, such a high number of the children in this study – 16 of 20 – had existing middle ear problems at the beginning of the study. Further, 25% of the individuals had elevated TSH but were untreated.

In the results of the study, according to the assessment tools used by the researchers, all of the participants scored less than the very first percentile. When this occurs, you would normally think that the investigators would have examined their assessment ranges. In this study the range for assessment seems to be very unreasonable as not one of the subjects could get to the first level, so how can you use this tool to measure improvement?

By way of analogy, the approach adopted by these researchers can be compared to a study assessing the strength of a group of participants by seeing how much weight they can lift. You then give them a series of 1 to 100 pound weights and not one person in the study can even lift the one pound weight. Perhaps – if you were genuinely interested in measuring the weight-lifting ability of your subjects.– you would reassess your measurement scale, and set out to measure at lower levels and in small increments.

It is interesting to note in this study, modest I.Q. increases were clustered among the younger subjects, whereas I.Q. decreases were more prevalent in the older subjects.

## 6. ELLIS ET AL[13]

Number of subjects: 10 adults with Down Syndrome

Ages: 21 to 40

Subjects given: Megavitamins according to Dr. Harrell's formula, 7 month duration

Study design: Double blinded study

Result: No significant benefits

Other commentary: Using 10 adults in an institutionalized setting speaks for itself.

I do not know if the poorly designed study by Dr. Harrell created a benefit or harm for the case for nutrients in Down Syndrome. The problem was that this was a poorly designed initial study using excessive vitamins, with a poor duration, improper age and poor numbers – but it had a positive result. This led to a flurry of studies whose sole objective was the null hypothesis – that is, studies that set out to disprove Harrell's hypothesis.

My bias is quite clear. I believe that non-megadose nutrients in doses which have been proven safe given at ages less than 2 years may improve cognitive function in Down Syndrome. The study disproving this notion has also not yet been done. The best study of mega-dose vitamins in Down Syndrome actually demonstrated a significant measurement in some aspects of I.Q. (Smith) but again was not reported because this was not relevant for disproving or disproving this notion of overall I.Q. as reported by the Harrell study.

A dramatic benefit in I.Q. with supplements in young infants was seen in the British Medical Journal study, but this was done in premature infants, not in infants with Down Syndrome. This well designed, controlled study is a bench mark for investigation of I.Q. in children. No study in Down Syndrome has approached the numbers, ages and length of time that this study has.

# The Piracetam study

The drug piracetam has become an issue in Down Syndrome due to the publicity it received on the ABC *Day One* show, where proponents of the drug claimed that piracetam had dramatic benefits in Down Syndrome.

The studies on piracetam involved its use with patients with Alzheimer's disease,[14] and it was also used successfully to treat dyslexia in children with an extremely safe risk profile.[15] From these studies, it appears that piracetam may have a benefit and it would appear to have very little risk. I spoke to the medical director of UCB Pharma (the manufacturers of piracetam). He thought it was interesting to use piracetam with children with Down Syndrome, but the effects were very mild compared to other drugs the company had in development for mental decline.

Unfortunately, the claims made about the benefits of a drug such as piracetam in Down Syndrome can also influence those who set out to study the drug. In yet another example of the implications of study bias, researchers then design studies that are geared only to picking up dramatic benefits, so more modest benefits might be missed in this all or nothing approach.

## Dr. Harrell's formula

The formula used by Dr. Harrell consisted of the following:

| | |
|---|---|
| Vitamin A palmitate | 15,000 IU |
| Vitamin D (cholacalciferol) | 300 IU |
| Thiamin mononitrate | 300 mg |
| Riboflavin | 200 mg |
| Niacinamide | 750 mg |
| Calcium pantothenate | 490 mg |
| Pyridoxine hydrochloride | 350 mg |
| Cobalamin | 1,000 ug |
| Folic acid | 400 ug |
| Vitamin C (ascorbic acid) | 1,500 mg |
| Vitamin E (d-a-tocopheryl succinate) | 600 IU |
| Magnesium (oxide) | 300 mg |
| Calcium (carbonate) | 400 mg |
| Zinc (oxide) | 30 mg |
| Manganese (gluconate) | 3 mg |
| Copper (gluconate) | 1.75 mg |
| Iron (ferrous fumarate) | 7.5 mg |
| Calcium phosphate (CaHPO4) | 37.5 mg |
| Iodide (KI) | 0.15 mg |

**Down Syndrome and Vitamin Therapy**

The only recent study on piracetam in Down Syndrome was done in Toronto, Canada in 2001.[16] It was conducted with 18 children with Down Syndrome, and designed to allow detection of large performance differences between the piracetam and placebo phases. A large effect size was chosen because most reports in the popular press have indicated immediate and substantive effects in children with Down Syndrome. In using a small number of subjects and a short duration of treatment (4 months), it is clear that the study was designed to only pick up dramatic differences.

Let's look at the results of the study. The study showed one significant benefit on piracetam: the stroop attention task, which is a measure of attention was significantly improved. This was the only one of 14 objective tests that showed significant improvement using piracatem. The other tests referenced in the study were subjective, based on parent and teacher questionnaires. There were seven types of questionnaires given, and six of the seven yielded significant results. Parents and teachers reported improvements in leadership, fewer thought problems, children seemed happier, there was fewer internalizing of problems and fewer total problems while taking piracetam. Interestingly, 11 of 18 parents commented that their child had improved cognition and attention while on piracetam.

There was only one negative effect of piracetam reported. There was noted to be poor attention while taking piracetam and side effects in 7 of 18 children, mostly associated with central nervous stimulatory system.

I must say that even for someone used to examining studies, such as myself, this is a confusing study. This is simply because the conclusion of the study does not match what actually occurred in the study. The written conclusion of the study was that piracetam does not enhance cognitive function in children with Down Syndrome. However, if you look at the study itself, that is not the conclusion. The following is a summary of what was reported in the study:

- One of 14 measures in a very short term (4 months) showed significant improvement in cognitive function.
- 5 of 7 teacher/parent questionnaires showed significant benefits on piracetam.
- Side effects were modest and related to excess stimulation.

All this in a study which was initially set up to disprove any benefit to piracetam with such a low number of participants in such a short time and only noting dramatic benefits. And after all this you CANNOT conclude that piracetam does not enhance cognitive function in children with Down Syndrome. If a drug company had been paying for this study, the conclusion would have been completely the opposite: they would have reported that piracetam DOES enhance cognitive function in children with Down Syndrome.

What is very disturbing about the significant benefits on the parent teacher questionnaires was that the researchers simply discounted them because they thought that the differences would be clinically insignificant although statistically significant.

## Studies by Chandra and Peeters-Ney

Let's take a look at two other studies with important implications for Down Syndrome. The first is by Dr. Chandra. This study measured baseline immune system and immune system responses following supplementation with vitamins, measured against the number of sick days in an elderly population.[17] He noted that over the period of one year, nutrient status and immunological status were assessed at baseline and frequency of illness due to infection was determined. The reason I feel this is a relevant study is that Chandra conducted a controlled trial using senior citizens, who as a segment of the population have traditionally suppressed immune systems. Chandra's study showed a 50% reduction in sick days, an improvement in white blood cells (natural killer cells) and increased interluken 2 and antibody response. Chandra's study is relevant because it gives us a model for an approach in studying nutrients in Down Syndrome, that is, by counting sick days. Chandra also notes very specifically that in previous studies, large pharmaceutical doses of a single nutrients were used. This approach violates the basic principles of nutrition and biochemistry, in that nutrients are interdependent. These dramatic benefits noted by Chandra in his study were as a result of using nutrients in doses much smaller than Harrell's mega-vitamin formula.

In the second study, Dr. Marie Peeters-Ney designed an observational study using the MSB formula with respect to sick days.[18] Our objective in this study was to show long-term benefits to the immune system and to correlate the benefits of immune system to specific nutrient levels. To this end, we have set up a full scale laboratory to measure these nutrient levels. We hope to set up more studies, as the initial results are similar to those obtained by Chandra, and to use our lab to determine these specific nutrient levels.

## Pharmaceutical studies versus vitamin studies

My objective in this area of vitamin research and studies and, for that matter, in this book is to make sure that especially in the area of Down Syndrome, none of the avenues of enquiry are closed as a result of study bias. Bias in study construction and reporting closes doors, because researchers fail to follow up, presuming that the answer has already been found.

Contrast this with the world of pharmaceutical drugs where the door is never closed – even when extravagant claims of benefit have been made in one instance and in the next instance the drug has been shown to be harmful if not deadly. The research never stops searching for the next new hot drug.

It must be said that the field of vitamin research has been tarnished by unnecessarily extravagant claims by some proponents of vitamins. But the fact is that many extravagant claims are made about drug therapies as well. The difference is that it's common for articles on vitamins to focus on criticizing these extravagant claims, and thereby cast doubt on the more moderate claims and proven – though somewhat more modest – benefits of vitamins. Rarely are articles on drug therapies framed this way. In articles on drug therapies, there are rarely mentions or references to the negative history of the particular drugs, even if its history was one of significant harm.

## Closing comments from Kent:

*At a recent Down Syndrome conference at which I was speaking, another speaker (who held a PhD in nutrition) stated that vitamin A is not an issue in Down Syndrome, because Dr. Pueschel had proven this. I asked the speaker if he had actually read Dr. Pueschel's study. He had not. I asked him whether he knew in detail what the study actually proved. He did not. So I told him what the study proved: water-soluble vitamin A (which is not found in nature or in any food and which is engineered to maximize absorption) is absorbed as efficiently by children with Down Syndrome as it is by children who do not have Down Syndrome – provided, of course, that you exclude from your study any children with Down Syndrome who have thyroid, bowel problems or celiac disease, which are proven to interfere with vitamin absorption. They do have significantly depressed distribution and metabolism of vitamin A in this study. So goes the world of research! – K.M.*

# Endnotes:

1. "Is Academic Medicine for Sale?" *New England Journal of Medicine* 2000; 342: 1516-1518

2. Friedberg M., et al. (1999) "Evaluation of conflict of interest in economic analyses of new drugs used in oncology." *Journal of the American Medical Association* 282: 1453-1457.

3. "Is Academic Medicine for Sale?" *New England Journal of Medicine* 2000; 342: 1516-1518

4. Wazana, A. (2000) "Physicians and the pharmaceutical industry: is a gift ever just a gift?" *Journal of the American Medical Association* 283:373-380.

5. Pueschel, S., et al. (1990) "Vitamin A gastrointestinal absorption in person's with Down's syndrome." *Journal of Mental Deficiency Research* 34: 269-75.

6. Pueschel, S. (1999) "Gastrointestinal concerns and nutritional issues in person's with Down's syndrome." *Down Syndrome Quarterly* 4(4): 1-11.

7. Lucas, A., et al. (1998) "Randomised trial of early diet in preterm babies and later intelligence quotient." *British Medical Journal* 317: 1481-7.

8. Weathers, C. (1983) "Effects of Nutritional Supplementation on IQ and Certain Other Variables Associated with Down Syndrome." *American Journal of Mental Deficiency* 88(2): 214-217.

9. Harrell, R.F., et al. (1981) "Can nutritional supplements help mentally retarded children? An exploratory study." *Proceedings of the National Academy of Sciences USA* 78: 574-578.

10. Coburn, S.P., et al. (1983) "Effect of megavitamin treatment on mental performance and plasma vitamin B6 concentrations in mentally retarded young adults." *American Journal of Clinical Nutrition* 38: 352-353

11. Smith, G., et al. (1984) "Use of megadoses of vitamins with minerals in Down syndrome. Journal of Pediatrics 105: 228-234.

12. Bennett, F.C., et al. (1983) Vitamin and Mineral Supplementation in Down's Syndrome." *Pediatrics* 72: 707-13.

13. Ellis, N. & Tomporowski, P. (1983) "Vitamin/Mineral Supplements and Intelligence of Institutionalized Mentally Retarded Adults." *American Journal of Mental Deficiency* 88(2): 211-4

14. Aguglia, E., et al. (1995) "Comparison of teniloxazine and piracetam in Alzheimer-type or vascular dementia." *Current Therapeutic Research* 56: 250-57.; Growdon, J.H., et al (1986) "Piracetam combined with lecithin in the treatment of Alzheimer's disease." *Neurobiology of Aging* 7: 269-76.

15. Wilsher, C.R., et al. (1987) "Piracetam and dyslexia: effects on reading tests." *Journal of Clinical Psychopharmacology.* 7: 230-37.; Ackerman, P.T., et al. (1991) "A trial of piracetam in two subgroups of students with dyslexia enrolled in summer tutoring." *Journal of Learning Disabilities* 24: 542-549.

16. Lobaugh, N.J., et al. (2001) "Piracetam therapy does not enhance cognitive functioning in children with Down syndrome." *Archives of Pediatric and Adolescent Medicine* 155: 442-48.

17. Chandra, R. (1992) "Effect of vitamin and trace-element supplementation on immune responses and infection in elderly subjects." *Lancet* 340: 1124-27

18. Peeters, M., and MacLeod, K. (1999) Unpublished data. Reviewed in *Bridges* 4(1).

# APPENDIX B

# GLOSSARY

**AMINO ACIDS**: Known as the "building blocks" of life, amino acids are critically important. Protein in the food we eat is broken down into amino acids. The body then builds the proteins it needs as part of every cell in our bodies. Some amino acids are also involved as neurotransmitters which carry nerve impulses from one cell to another. In other words, they're needed to send and receive messages from the brain. Other amino acids work helping vitamins and minerals to function. Some amino acids are called non-essential. What this really means (because they ARE essential) is that they can be made in our body. The remaining (called essential) have to come from our food or from supplements.

**ANEMIA**: Insufficient number of red blood cells or hemoglobin in blood.

**ANTIBODY** (also known as **IMMUNOGLOBULIN**): proteins produced by white blood cells that attach to antigens and disable them

**ANTIGEN**: foreign invaders (bacteria, virus, toxin)

**BACTERIA**: Single-celled organisms that are found in food, air, soil and the human body. Good bacteria prevent infections. Other bacteria cause disease.

**BOWEL**: The gastrointestinal system of the body extending from the stomach to the anal opening. Includes small intestine (composed of the duodenum, jejunum, and ileum) and colon (large intestine).

**CASE REPORT STUDY**: descriptive reports of a single patient's case history outlining treatments and outcome

**CHROMOSOMES**: The genetic material present in cells is in the form of chromosomes. Human cells have 46 chromosomes in two sets of 23 pairs. Genes are portions of chromosomes.

**CLINICAL TRIAL**: participants are given some intervention, for example a drug, and then followed up for any outcomes

**CROSSOVER STUDY**: subjects receive both the intervention and control treatments in random order, often with periods without treatment in between

**CYSTATHIONINE-BETA SYNTHASE (CBS)**: gene located on the 21st chromosome with coding for production of the CBS protein which acts as an enzyme in chain reaction conversion of amino aciDown Syndrome: homocysteine to cystathionine to cysteine, a precursor to glutathione (necessary to protect liver and brain from toxic substances)

**DNA (DEOXYRIBONUCLEIC ACID)**: chemical inside cell nucleus carrying genetic instructions for production of living organisms (DNA in genes is constantly mutating and being repaired)

**DOUBLE BLIND STUDY**: neither subjects nor investigators knew who was receiving what treatment

**ENZYMES AND COENZYMES**: An enzyme is a protein that helps chemical reactions work. A coenzyme is a molecule (like a vitamin or mineral) that helps the enzyme work better. Enzymes are also referred to as the "sparks of life." These biological substance are made up of proteins and act as catalysts. They are essential for digesting food, stimulating the brain, providing cellular energy and repairing all tissues, organs and cells.

**FATTY ACIDS**: organic acids found in fats and oils

**FOLATE**: functions as a single carbon donor in synthesis of DNA; needed for production of red blood cells, tissue growth and cell function

**FOLIC ACID**: synthetic form of folate found in supplements or added to foods

**FUNGI**: Multi-cellular microorganisms that are universally distributed and include molds, mushrooms, mildews. Some are harmful to plants and animals, including humans, while some fungi are valued as food or for the fermentations that they produce (for example yeast and beer).

**HEMOGLOBIN**: Red pigment in blood that combines with oxygen to produce cellular energy

**HOMOCYSTEINE**: amino acid made from methionine that in turn converts into other amino acids

**HORMONES**: Biological substances made up of proteins and used to regulate body functions such as growth and metabolism.

**HYDROGEN**: key component of many biological/organic molecules in our bodies; can also be a very powerful free radical

**HYDROGENATION**: process of oxidation that turns liquid fat into solid fat by saturating it (heating) with hydrogen

**IN VIVO**: in the living organism

**IN VITRO**: in the laboratory

**LYMPH**: fluid that carries nutrients from blood to cells and returns waste from cells to blood

**LYMPHOCYTE**: a type of white blood cell divided into two categories: B cells which are made in the bone marrow and produce antibodies; T cells which mature in the thymus and attack invading organisms

**MACROCYTOSIS**: Increase in red blood cell size due to inability to divide because DNA synthesis has been disturbed

**MEAN CORPUSCULAR VOLUME (MCV)**: test that measures macrocytosis

**METABOLISM**: chemical reactions that take place in the cells of the body; includes breakdown of organic compounds to yield energy (catabolism) and synthesis of materials from simpler substances (anabolism).

**METHYL GROUP**: One unit of carbon (basic element from which all organic matter is created) combined with three units of hydrogen; essential in production of DNA

**OXYGEN**: required for breathing; essential element that is a key component of many biological/organic molecules in our bodies; extremely chemically active

**OXIDATION**: when an atom or molecule loses electrons, it is oxidized; (i.e. when an antioxidant steals an electron from a fat, the fat has been oxidized)

**POLYUNSATURATED FATS**: fats saturated with two or more hydrogen atoms

**PROTEIN**: A macronutrient, like fat and carbohydrates, that provides energy for the body. Proteins are digested in the gastrointestinal tract and broken down into amino acids. The amino acids are then used to form new proteins in the body. Protein-rich substances in our body include muscle, blood, ligaments, skin, internal organs, glands, nails and hair. Enzymes, hormones and antibodies are also composed of protein.

**RANDOMIZED CONTROLLED STUDY**: participants are chosen at random from among a larger group; each group receives a different intervention (including a placebo) then both groups are studied for outcome. This type of study aims to have identical groups at the outset so that the only difference, the treatment administered, can be attributed for any differences in outcome.

**S-ADENOSYLMETHIONINE (SAM)**: the active methyl donor that is a vital part of countless metabolic reactions throughout the body.

**SAM CYCLE**: a cycle that helps transport methyl groups

**SATURATED FATS**: solid fats that have all their carbon atoms saturated with hydrogen

**SINGLE BLIND STUDY**: subjects did not know what treatment they were receiving

**UNSATURATED FATS**: liquid fats with empty spaces because of missing hydrogen atoms

**VIRUS**: Infectious, disease-causing particles that reproduce by invading and taking over living cells; virus is Latin for poison.

**WHITE BLOOD CELLS (LEUKOCYTES)**: Most important part of immune system consisting of many different types of cells that destroy bacteria and viruses

# NOTES